Discarded by
Millville Public Library

CANCER ETIOLOGY, DIAGNOSIS AND TREATMENTS

SARCOMA

SYMPTOMS, CAUSES AND TREATMENTS

CANCER ETIOLOGY, DIAGNOSIS AND TREATMENTS

Additional books in this series can be found on Nova's website under the Series tab.

Additional E-books in this series can be found on Nova's website under the E-book tab.

CANCER ETIOLOGY, DIAGNOSIS AND TREATMENTS

SARCOMA

SYMPTOMS, CAUSES AND TREATMENTS

ERIC J. BUTLER
EDITOR

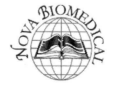

Nova Biomedical Books
New York

Copyright © 2012 by Nova Science Publishers, Inc.

All rights reserved. No part of this book may be reproduced, stored in a retrieval system or transmitted in any form or by any means: electronic, electrostatic, magnetic, tape, mechanical photocopying, recording or otherwise without the written permission of the Publisher.

For permission to use material from this book please contact us:
Telephone 631-231-7269; Fax 631-231-8175
Web Site: http://www.novapublishers.com

NOTICE TO THE READER

The Publisher has taken reasonable care in the preparation of this book, but makes no expressed or implied warranty of any kind and assumes no responsibility for any errors or omissions. No liability is assumed for incidental or consequential damages in connection with or arising out of information contained in this book. The Publisher shall not be liable for any special, consequential, or exemplary damages resulting, in whole or in part, from the readers' use of, or reliance upon, this material. Any parts of this book based on government reports are so indicated and copyright is claimed for those parts to the extent applicable to compilations of such works.

Independent verification should be sought for any data, advice or recommendations contained in this book. In addition, no responsibility is assumed by the publisher for any injury and/or damage to persons or property arising from any methods, products, instructions, ideas or otherwise contained in this publication.

This publication is designed to provide accurate and authoritative information with regard to the subject matter covered herein. It is sold with the clear understanding that the Publisher is not engaged in rendering legal or any other professional services. If legal or any other expert assistance is required, the services of a competent person should be sought. FROM A DECLARATION OF PARTICIPANTS JOINTLY ADOPTED BY A COMMITTEE OF THE AMERICAN BAR ASSOCIATION AND A COMMITTEE OF PUBLISHERS.

Additional color graphics may be available in the e-book version of this book.

Library of Congress Cataloging-in-Publication Data

Sarcoma : symptoms, causes, and treatments / editor, Eric J. Butler.
    p. ; cm.
Includes bibliographical references and index.
ISBN 978-1-62100-362-5 (hardcover)
I. Butler, Eric J.
[DNLM: 1. Sarcoma. QZ 345]
LC classification not assigned
616.99'4--dc23
                    2011033363

Published by Nova Science Publishers, Inc. † New York

Contents

Preface		**vii**
Chapter I	Sarcoma: Symptoms, Causes and Treatments *Mariangela Palladino*	1
Chapter II	Clinic-Histopathologic Diagnosis of the Kaposi's Sarcoma *Roberto Gabriel Albin and Juan Carlos Perez-Cárdenas*	35
Chapter III	M5076 Ovarian Sarcoma in Mice: Novel Chemotherapy by Drug Delivery System *Yasuyuki Sadzuka*	63
Chapter IV	Advances in Chondrosarcoma Treatment: Engineering in vitro Three-Dimensional Models *YuLong Han, LiHong Zhou, ShuQi Wang, JinHui Wu, ZhenFeng Duan, TianJian Lu and Feng Xu*	85
Chapter V	The Potential of Suicide Plus Immune Gene Therapy for Treating Osteosarcoma: The Experience on Canine Veterinary Patients *Liliana M. E. Finocchiaro, Agustina Spector, Ursula A. Rossi, María L. Gil-Cardeza, José L. Suarez, María D. Riveros, Marcela S. Villaverde and Gerardo C. Glikin*	107

Contents

Chapter VI	New Concept of Limb Salvage Surgery in Musculoskeletal Sarcomas with Acridine Orange Therapy *Katsuyuki Kusuzaki, Shigekuni Hosogi, Eishi Ashihara, Takao Matsubara, Haruhiko Satonaka, Tomoki Nakamura, Akihiko Matsumine, Akihiro Sudo, Atsumasa Uchida, Hiroaki Murata, Nicola Baldini, Stefano Fais and Yoshinori Marunaka*	123
Chapter VII	The Role of Surgery in Children with Head and Neck Rhabdomyosarcoma and Ewing's Sarcoma *P. Gradoni, D. Giordano, G. Oretti, M. Fantoni and T. Ferri*	139
Chapter VIII	Gastrointestinal Kaposi's Sarcoma: Diagnosis and Clinical Features *Naoyoshi Nagata, Ryo Nakashima, Sou Nishimura, Naoki Asayma, Kazuhiro Watanabe, Koh Imbe, Tomoyuki Yada, Junichi Akiyama, Hirohisa Yazaki, Shinichi Oka and Naomi Uemura*	153
Index		167

Preface

Sarcomas are a group of rare malignant tumors that constitute less than 1% of all cancers, arising from the mesenchymal system. About 80% originate in soft tissue (muscle, nerves, joints, blood vessels, deep skin tissues, and fat), while the remainder originate in bone and cartilage. In this book, the authors present topical research on the symptoms, causes and treatments of sarcoma. Some of the topics discussed include clinical-histopathologic diagnosis of the kaposi's sarcoma; ovarian sarcoma in mice; advances in chondrosarcoma treatment; the potential of suicide plus immune gene therapy for treating osteosarcoma; new concepts of limb salvage surgery in musculoskeletal sarcomas with acridine orange therapy; the role of surgery in children with head and neck rhabdomyosarcoma and gastrointestinal kaposi's sarcoma.

Chapter 1 - Sarcomas are a group of rare malignant tumors that constitute less than 1% of all cancers, arising from the mesenchymal system. About 80% originate in soft tissue (muscle, nerves, joints, blood vessels, deep skin tissues, and fat), while the remainder originate in bone and cartilage. Approximately, 10,520 new cases of soft-tissue sarcoma and 2,650 new cases of bone sarcoma have been diagnosed in the USA in 2010.

There are more than 50 histological subtypes of soft tissue sarcomas recognized by the World Health Organization. The most common types are leiomyosarcoma, malignant fibrous histiocytoma and liposarcoma. Osteosarcoma is the most common type of bone sarcomas, followed by chondrosarcoma and Ewing sarcoma.

The etiology of most malignant sarcomas is unknown. Rarely, predisposing factors such as genetic susceptibility, radiation therapy, chemotherapy, preexisting benign tumors, viral infection, immunodeficiency, traumatic events and orthopedic implants, have been found related with the development of bone and soft tissue malignancies.

Soft tissue tumor often presents as a painless, incidentally discovered mass, that does not limit function. Most soft tissue superficial neoformations are benign, while all deep located lesions are likely to be malignant. Bone sarcomas usually present with localized pain and swelling, sometimes with associated erythema. Constitutional symptoms are rare in patients with bone or soft-tissue sarcomas.

Standard radiography is useful for characterizing osseous neoformations, but has a very limited role in the identification of soft-tissue sarcomas. Ultrasonography has a limited value in the diagnosis and follow-up of soft-tissue sarcomas, while is not effective in the evaluation of bone lesions, as sound waves are unable to penetrate the bony cortex. Magnetic resonance imaging represents the standard choice for evaluation of most lesions, while computed tomography is particular important for evaluation of metastatic disease. Positron emission tomography technique allows detection of tumor metabolic activity rather than tumor size, so it appears more sensitive than topographical techniques. Further, a *biopsy* is an essential part of the work-up, as it allows to identify the type of tumor and to provide information about the future treatment protocol.

The prognosis of sarcomas correlates with histological grade. Low-grade sarcomas are unlikely to metastasize, therefore surgical excision with negative tissue margins in all directions is usually the standard treatment option. High-grade sarcomas have a high metastatic potential and needs to be treated with chemotherapy or radiation. Moreover, chemotherapy or radiation may be used as neoadjuvant therapy prior to surgery.

Chapter 2 - The Kaposi's Sarcoma (KS) has acquired a relevant clinical importance in the past 20 years because it is a malignant tumor frequently associated with HIV infection. It is a multifocal vascular lesion of low-grade malignancy that typically appears on the skin of the lower extremities. The internal organs and lymph nodes are damaged less frequently. More rarely involve muscles, the Central Nervous System, peripheral nerves, heart, breast, salivary glands and the eyes. Approximately 60% of the KS are presented with purple nodular lesions on the skin and/or of the oral mucosa. The other 40% has visceral injury with involvement of the gastrointestinal tract or invasion of the lungs. The disease can take in these cases with bleeding, perforations and obstruction. When there is a commitment to gastrointestinal tract, endoscopic study shows purple nodular lesions characteristic on the way from the mucosa. The differential diagnosis includes the hemangioma, bacillary angiomatosis,

Blue Rubber Bleb Nevus Syndrome, the Osler-Weber-Rendu disease, Klippel-Trenaunay Syndrome and von Hippel-Lindau disease. That is why we need an accurate histopathological diagnosis in order to confirm the KS. The Immunohistochemistry staining for the virus HHV-8 have a 95-98% sensitivity and 100% specificity for the KS lesions. Other studies of Immunohistochemistry do not less important are the staining for CD31, CD34, CD40, Ki67, alpha Actin (SMA) and D2-40. The purpose of this chapter is to highlight the importance of maintaining a high clinical suspicion of the disease when the doctor faced with symptoms and signs that is studying the disease. On the other hand, the doctor must know the different diagnostic tools that are currently in clinical pathology in order to confirm this disease and thus engage in misdiagnosis, due the implications for the physical and mental health to which leads to the confirmation of the diagnosis of the KS. The authors intend to encourage the learning of all the clinical syndromes of presentation of the KS as well as the importance of the accurate diagnosis by immunohistochemical methods.

Chapter 3 - M5076 ovarian sarcoma is transplantable murine reticulum sarcoma originating in ovary of C57BL/6 mice and highly invasive and metastatic. When M5076 ovarian sarcoma is s.c. transplanted onto the backs of mice, solid tumor arises, spontaneously metastasizes to the liver and lung, and then kills the mice within about 25-30 days. This sarcoma exhibited lower sensitivity to antitumor agent as doxorubicin (DOX). Namely, M5076 ovarian sarcoma which has high metastasis and resistance, induced unfavorable prognosis on host body. In current chemotherapy, it is important for treatment on the sarcoma of these profiles.

On biochemical modulation, the pharmacodynamics of antitumor agent is modulated by combination with another drug in order to enhance the antitumor activity or to reduce the adverse reaction, the chemotherapic index is thereby enhanced. From these points, this concept is considered as drug delivery system. Theanine is specific amino acid and umami component in green tea. Theanine does not have antitumor activity whereas enhance some antitumor agents induced efficacy. Namely, the combination of theanine with non-effective dose of doxorubicin (DOX) suppressed M5076 ovarian sarcoma growing in vivo. In vitro, theanine inhibited DOX efflux from M5076 ovarian sarcoma cell and in vivo, combined theanine increased DOX concentration in the tumor without no change of DOX concentration in normal tissues in sarcoma bearing mice. From the evaluation in detail, the mechanism for the theanine induced effects speculated as follows. Some of the DOX taken up by M5076 ovarian sarcoma cells binds to glutathione (GSH) and thereby generates the GS-DOX conjugate. The conjugate is released extracellularly by the GS-X pump on M5076 ovarian sarcoma cells. Theanine suppressed the uptake of glutamate through inhibitions of GLAST and GLT-1 as glutamate transporters and thereafter reduced the biosynthesis of GSH in sarcoma cells. Then, generation of the conjugate of intracellular DOX and GSH is affected and the release of the GS-DOX conjugate by sarcoma cells via the MRP5/GS-X pump decrease.

On M5076 ovarian sarcoma cells, anserine and taurine as dipeptide, glutamate transporter inhibitors and methylxanthine derivatives enhanced antitumor activity of DOX, too. In conclusion, it is expected that the combination of food components and other agent with antitumor agent advances novel therapy on some sarcomas.

Chapter 4 - Chondrosarcoma is a common bone cancer that affects thousands of people worldwide. Although chondrosarcoma has been recognized for a long time, little breakthrough has been achieved in the treatment. Currently, surgery is the only effective treatment, despite the fact that it negatively affects the patient's life quality and has high risks of recurrence. To address this, various treatment regimens based on radiotherapy and chemotherapy have been developed, which however showed limited success due to the cancer's resistance to radiotherapy and chemotherapy. This clinical situation can be improved by further understanding on cancer-treatment interactions, which depends on the availability of clinically relevant *in vitro* models. However, existing cancer models are mainly based on two-dimensional (2D) culture, which has shown significantly different behaviors compared to native three-dimensional (3D) cancer tissues. Emerging novel biomaterials (e.g., hydrogels) and tissue engineering methods offer great potential to address these challenges. In this chapter, the authors present state-of-the-art advances in chondrosarcoma treatment and *in vitro* cancer models, with focus on engineering 3D cell microenvironment. These achievements may lead to the foundation of basic research and bridge the gap between lab research and clinical treatment.

Chapter 5 - Comparative oncology amalgamates the experience on naturally occurring cancers in veterinary patients into more general studies of cancer, especially those focused on the human disease. Naturally occurring tumors in dogs have clinical and biological similarities to human cancers that are difficult to replicate in other model systems.

Osteosarcoma (OSA) accounts for approximately 85% of primary bone cancers in the dog. It is a common cancer of large to giant breed dogs, and it occurs primarily in the appendicular skeleton. Being a common and highly metastatic tumor, it does not have additional treatment options when adjuvant chemotherapy has failed against its disseminated form. Even with removal of the primary tumor, before spread of the cancer is clinically detectable, metastases to lung, bone, or other sites eventually develop in almost all dogs. Palliative radiation therapy for bone pain is indicated in those dogs that do not undergo amputation or a limb-sparing surgery. Standard treatments result in median survival rates ranging between 78 and 130 days.

In such context the need to develop new treatments to fight OSA is compelling. While most of cancer gene therapy for canine veterinary patients was aimed to spontaneous melanoma and some to primary canine soft-tissue sarcomas, only one was specifically aimed to OSA. Therefore, the authors propose a new treatment combining: (i) the local antiproliferative effects of interferon-β and HSV-thymidine kinase suicide gene therapy with (ii) the systemic effects triggered by OSA antigens in an immunostimulatory environment created by the slow secretion of granulocyte and macrophage colony-stimulating factor and interleukin-2.

Beyond the high safety standard of the proposed treatment on six canine osteosarcoma patients, four of them survived more than 6 months (among them, two exceeded 1 year). In addition, the treatment prevented or delayed local relapse, regional metastases and distant metastases, suggesting a strong systemic antitumor immunity.

The authors are presenting detailed evidences of two cases of a very successful outcome: (i) a first one presenting a long term recurrence-free period after tumor surgical excision and (ii) a second one of a long-lasting complete remission without surgical intervention.

As a conclusion of this work the authors suggest that the use of this treatment, associated or not to the surgical removal of the tumor (depending on the initial stage of the disease), would be safe and could delay or prevent recurrence and metastases, with the consequent quality of life and survival rate improvement. To establish the treatment efficacy, the encouraging results presented here warrant the proposal of a subsequent trial including a representative amount of canine patients.

Chapter 6 - Although limb salvage surgery involving wide resection and limb reconstruction for musculoskeletal sarcomas is well established for low risk of local tumor recurrence, limb function is unsatisfactory for many patients because of the disability in active athletics such as running, jumping, throwing, swimming etc. To avoid poor limb function caused by surgery, it is important to preserve normal nerves, vessels, bones, joints and muscles adjacent to tumor as possible as we can, supported by effective adjuvant therapy to inhibit local tumor recurrence.

To develop minimally-invasive limb salvage surgery with minimal damage of normal tissues and low risk of local recurrence, the authors have recently established a new limb salvage modality of acridine orange (AO) therapy (AOT) based on photodynamic surgery (PDS), photodynamic therapy (PDT) and radiodynamic therapy (RDT) using AO in patients with high-grade malignant musculoskeletal sarcoma. Clinical outcomes of the study showed that: 1) low risk of local recurrence which is almost the same as that with conventional wide resection, and 2) superior limb function to that by wide resection.

In this chapter, the authors present mechanisms of cytocidal effects of AOT based on experimental research and clinical outcome of AOT applied to musculoskeletal sarcoma patients.

Chapter 7 - Rhabdomyosarcoma (RMS) is a soft tissue malignant neoplasm and it is the most common paediatric solid tumour. Ewing's sarcoma (ES) is a primary bone malignant neoplasm and it is the second most common primary malignant tumour of bone found in children after osteosarcoma. These tumours are uncommon in adults: RMS follows a bimodal distribution, with peak incidence between 2 and 4 years and between 12 and 16 years. Ewing's sarcoma has a peak incidence during the second decade of life. Head and neck localizations are frequent in RMS, accounting for 35-40% of the cases while they are rare in ES (1-4%).

Rhabdomyosarcoma and ES share some crucial biologic and clinical features: they are high grade tumours with local aggressiveness and strong potential to metastasize; both tumours are considered "systemic diseases" given the rapid development of metastatic spread. Because of that, systemic chemotherapy plays an essential role in treating distant metastases regardless their identification at initial staging; unlike other soft tissue sarcomas and osteogenic sarcoma, RMS and ES are relatively sensitive to chemotherapy and radiotherapy; in other sarcomas there are no good alternative to radical surgery; standard treatment for RMS and ES is a multimodal therapy involving chemotherapy, radiotherapy and surgery; until 1991, patients with extraosseous ES were eligible for the Intergroup Rhabdomyosarcoma Study (IRS) protocols.

Prior to the introduction of antineoplastic drugs, surgery played the central role in the cure of patients with RMS and ES; in the last four decades, the development of multi-agent chemotherapy protocols resulted in a significant improvement in long-term survival: from 25% (RMS) and 10% (ES) in 1970, to approximately 70% nowadays. Such scenario has leaded to a critical discussion in literature concerning the role of surgical treatment. Particular surgical challenge is represented by tumours affecting the head and neck. These anatomical sites do not generally lend themselves to a radical surgical approach as a primary procedure; complete resection is not feasible in many patients and, even if possible, is unlikely to be achieved without major functional or cosmetic consequences. Nevertheless, radical surgery is still considered the best choice to obtain the local control. Very few studies have been focused on the feasibility and effectiveness of surgical resection. Defined criteria to establish the risks and the benefits of surgical treatment do not exist at this time. Despite the improvement in diagnostic techniques, especially imaging, some authors acknowledge that incomplete surgical excision may be due to inadequate preoperative evaluation. Given the rarity of these neoplasms, most studies deal with relatively small surgical series or even case reports; indications evidently arise from personal experiences and many authors conclude that the surgical treatment should be decided on a case by case basis.

In order to delineate the role of surgery in head and neck RMS and ES, indications, feasibility and timing criteria of surgical treatment have been reviewed and extracted from literature. The management of orbital RMS is unique because surgery does not confer any advantage over chemotherapy and radiotherapy in terms of survival, thus it won't be discussed herein

Chapter 8 - *Background*: Kaposi's sarcoma (KS) is a rare malignant tumor, but often occurs in patients with AIDS. The gastrointestinal (GI) tract is the third most commonly affected site after the skin and the lymph nodes. Early diagnosis of GI-KS is important because advanced GI lesions may cause hemorrhage, perforation, and obstruction. However, the clinical characteristics of GI-KS have not been fully studied. The aim of this study was to clarify the key clinical factors for the diagnosis of GI-KS.

Methods: The authors retrospectively reviewed the cases of 311 HIV-infected patients who had undergone endoscopy between 2003 and 2007. Endoscopic images of tissue biopsies and supplementary immunological staining were used in the diagnosis of GI-KS. Clinical parameters such as HIV infection route, fecal occult blood test (FOBT) results, GI symptoms, CD4 lymphocyte count, and the viral load of KS-associated herpes virus (KSHV) in the blood were assessed. Skin lesions and extracutaneous spread of KS were examined prior to endoscopy.

Results: Twenty-seven of the 311 patients had a diagnosis of GI-KS. Endoscopic biopsy was performed on a total of 238 lesions suspected to be GI-KS, of these, 162 lesions (68.1%) were confirmed to be GI-KS. Common organ involvement in the GI-KS patients was the stomach (11 patients), duodenum (10), colon (7), esophagus (4), rectum (3), and terminal ileum (2). Age and sex were not significant factors but CD4 count was significantly lower in patients with GI-KS than those without GI-KS (median KS+ 69 vs. KS- 270.5, $p<0.01$).

Among 27 patients with GI-KS, men who have sex with men (MSM) was the most frequent HIV infection route in patients with GI-KS (21/27). FOBT was positive in 17% of cases involving the upper GI tract and in 30% of those involving the lower intestinal tract. GI symptoms were observed in 19%. KSHV viral loads were positive in 50%, and the median level was 900 copy/ml. Other organs involvement of KS were the skin (23), lymph nodes (15), oral cavity (4), respiratory tract (3), conjunctiva (2), and liver (1). In 4 patients, all asymptomatic MSM patients, KS lesions were found only in the GI tract.

Conclusion: Upper endoscopy should be considered for patients especially with particularly low CD4 counts who are MSM even when patients are asymptomatic or FOBT results are negative. Several biopsies with immunohistochemical staining are recommended for pathological confirmation. This strategy can lead to early diagnosis and treatment of GI-KS.

In: Sarcoma ISBN: 978-1-62100-362-5
Editor: Eric J. Butler © 2012 Nova Science Publishers, Inc.

Chapter I

Sarcoma: Symptoms, Causes and Treatments

Mariangela Palladino

Department of Hematology, A. Gemelli University Hospital, Catholic University School of Medicine, Rome, Italy
Department of Medicine (Division of Cardiovascular Research), St. Elizabeth's Medical Center, Tufts University School of Medicine, Boston, MA, U. S.

Abstract

Sarcomas are a group of rare malignant tumors that constitute less than 1% of all cancers, arising from the mesenchymal system. About 80% originate in soft tissue (muscle, nerves, joints, blood vessels, deep skin tissues, and fat), while the remainder originate in bone and cartilage. Approximately, 10,520 new cases of soft-tissue sarcoma and 2,650 new cases of bone sarcoma have been diagnosed in the USA in 2010.

There are more than 50 histological subtypes of soft tissue sarcomas recognized by the World Health Organization. The most common types are leiomyosarcoma, malignant fibrous histiocytoma and liposarcoma. Osteosarcoma is the most common type of bone sarcomas, followed by chondrosarcoma and Ewing sarcoma.

The etiology of most malignant sarcomas is unknown. Rarely, predisposing factors such as genetic susceptibility, radiation therapy, chemotherapy, preexisting benign tumors, viral infection, immune-deficiency, traumatic events and orthopedic implants, have been found related with the development of bone and soft tissue malignancies.

Soft tissue tumor often presents as a painless, incidentally discovered mass, that does not limit function. Most soft tissue superficial neoformations are benign, while all deep located lesions are likely to be malignant. Bone sarcomas usually present with localized pain and swelling, sometimes with associated erythema. Constitutional symptoms are rare in patients with bone or soft-tissue sarcomas.

Standard radiography is useful for characterizing osseous neoformations, but has a very limited role in the identification of soft-tissue sarcomas. Ultrasonography has a limited value in the diagnosis and follow-up of soft-tissue sarcomas, while is not effective in the evaluation of bone lesions, as sound waves are unable to penetrate the bony cortex. Magnetic resonance imaging represents the standard choice for evaluation of most lesions, while computed tomography is particular important for evaluation of metastatic disease. Positron emission tomography technique allows detection of tumor metabolic activity rather than tumor size, so it appears more sensitive than topographical techniques. Further, a *biopsy* is an essential part of the work-up, as it allows to identify the type of tumor and to provide information about the future treatment protocol.

The prognosis of sarcomas correlates with histological grade. Low-grade sarcomas are unlikely to metastasize, therefore surgical excision with negative tissue margins in all directions is usually the standard treatment option. High-grade sarcomas have a high metastatic potential and needs to be treated with chemotherapy or radiation. Moreover, chemotherapy or radiation may be used as neoadjuvant therapy prior to surgery.

Introduction

Sarcomas are rare neoplasms arising from connective tissues. They are usually named for the type of tissue in which they begin. Two main groups can be distinguished: those derived from soft tissues and those derived from bone.

Soft Tissue Sarcomas

Soft tissue sarcomas (STSs) constitute a heterogeneous group of mesodermal tumors. The relative rarity and the varied and unusual presentation sometimes make diagnosis extremely difficult. Most STSs are benign, being the estimated ratio benign: malignant 100: 1. However, about one half of patients with diagnosis of malignant sarcoma will die from it [1].

Table 1. WHO classification of soft tissue tumors

ADIPOCYTIC TUMOURS	Giant cell angiofibroma
Benign	
Lipoma	Intermediate (locally aggressive)
Lipomatosis	Superficial fibromatoses (palmar/ plantar)
Lipomatosis of nerve	Desmoid-type fibromatoses
Lipoblastoma / Lipoblastomatosis	Lipofibromatosis
Angiolipoma	
Myolipoma	Intermediate (rarely metastasizing)
Chondroid lipoma	Solitary fibrous tumour
Extrarenal angiomyolipoma	and haemangiopericytoma
Extra-adrenal myelolipoma	(incl. lipomatous haemangiopericytoma)
Spindle cell/	Inflammatory myofibroblastic tumour
Pleomorphic lipoma	Low grade myofibroblastic sarcoma
Hibernoma	Myxoinflammatory
	fibroblastic sarcoma
Intermediate (locally aggressive)	Infantile fibrosarcoma
Atypical lipomatous tumour/	
Well differentiated liposarcoma	Malignant
	Adult fibrosarcoma
Malignant	Myxofibrosarcoma
Dedifferentiated liposarcoma	Low grade fibromyxoid sarcoma
Myxoid liposarcoma	hyalinizing spindle cell tumour
Round cell liposarcoma	Sclerosing epithelioid fibrosarcoma
Pleomorphic liposarcoma	
Mixed-type liposarcoma	SO-CALLED FIBROHISTIOCYTIC TUMOURS
Liposarcoma, not otherwise specified	Benign
	Giant cell tumour of tendon sheath
FIBROBLASTIC / MYOFIBROBLASTIC	Diffuse-type giant cell tumour
TUMOURS	Deep benign fibrous histiocytoma
Benign	
Nodular fasciitis	Intermediate (rarely metastasizing)
Proliferative fasciitis	Plexiform fibrohistiocytic tumour
Proliferative myositis	Giant cell tumour of soft tissues
Myositis ossificans	
fibro-osseous pseudotumour of digits	Malignant
Ischaemic fasciitis	Pleomorphic 'MFH' / Undifferentiated
Elastofibroma	pleomorphic sarcoma
Fibrous hamartoma of infancy	Giant cell 'MFH' / Undifferentiated
Myofibroma / Myofibromatosis	pleomorphic sarcoma
Fibromatosis colli	with giant cells
Juvenile hyaline fibromatosis	Inflammatory 'MFH' / Undifferentiated
Inclusion body fibromatosis	pleomorphic sarcoma with
Fibroma of tendon sheath	prominent inflammation
Desmoplastic fibroblastoma	
Mammary-type myofibroblastoma	
Calcifying aponeurotic fibroma	
Angiomyofibroblastoma	

Table 1. (Continued).

Cellular angiofibroma Nuchal-type fibroma Gardner fibroma Calcifying fibrous tumour **SMOOTH MUSCLE TUMORS** Angioleiomyoma Deep leiomyoma Genital leyomioma Leyomyosarcoma (excluding skin) **PERICYTIC (PERIVASCULAR) TUMOURS** Glomus tumour (and variants) malignant glomus tumour Myopericytoma **SKELETAL MUSCLE TUMOURS** Benign Rhabdomyoma adult type fetal type genital type Malignant Embryonal rhabdomyosarcoma (incl. spindle cell, botryoid, anaplastic) Alveolar rhabdomyosarcoma (incl. solid, anaplastic) Pleomorphic rhabdomyosarcoma **VASCULAR TUMOURS** Benign Haemangiomas of subcut/deep soft tissue: capillary cavernous arteriovenous venous intramuscular synovial Epithelioid haemangioma Angiomatosis Lymphangioma Intermediate (locally aggressive) Kaposiform haemangioendothelioma Intermediate (rarely metastasizing) Retiform haemangioendothelioma Papillary intralymphatic angioendothelioma Composite haemangioendothelioma Kaposi Sarcoma	Malignant Epithelioid haemangioendothelioma Angiosarcoma of soft tissue **CHONDRO-OSSEOUS TUMOURS** Soft tissue chondroma Mesenchymal chondrosarcoma Extraskeletal osteosarcoma **TUMOURS OF UNCERTAIN DIFFERENTIATION** Benign Intramuscular myxoma (incl. cellular variant) Juxta-articular myxoma Deep ('aggressive') angiomyxoma Pleomorphic hyalinizing angiectatic tumour Ectopic hamartomatous thymoma Intermediate (rarely metastasizing) Angiomatoid fibrous histiocytoma Ossifying fibromyxoid tumour (incl. atypical / malignant) Mixed tumour/ Myoepithelioma/ Parachordoma Malignant Synovial sarcoma Epithelioid sarcoma Alveolar soft part sarcoma Clear cell sarcoma of soft tissue Extraskeletal myxoid chondrosarcoma ("chordoid" type) PNET / Extraskeletal Ewing tumour pPNET extraskeletal Ewing tumour Desmoplastic small round cell tumour Extra-renal rhabdoid tumour Malignant mesenchymoma Neoplasms with perivascular epithelioid cell differentiation (PEComa) clear cell myomelanocytic tumour Intimal sarcoma

Incidence

STSs are relatively rare diseases, with estimated fewer than 5000 cases per annum in the United States [2], it is to say less than 1% of all neoplasms in the general population. In children, however, they constitute 6.5% of all cancers.

Epidemiology

All age groups are equally affected; about 15% are found in children < 15 years and 40% in adult after 55 years. Males have slightly higher incidence rates than females. There is no evidence for preferential geographic distributions, although slightly higher incidence rates in black children respect to white children have been evidenced, especially among children 15-19 years old [3, 4].

The three most common STSs are leiomyosarcoma, malignant fibrous histiocytoma (MFH), liposarcoma, fibrosarcoma, and synovial sarcoma. Approximately, leyomiosarcoma has an annual incidence rate of 12.2 cases per million population, MHF of 8.8 cases per million population, liposarcoma of 5.9 cases per million population, fibrosarcoma of 1.8 cases per million population, while synovial sarcoma of 1.1 case per million population [5]. Rhabdomyosarcoma is the most common STS among children 0-14 years old, representing almost 50% of STS for this age range, with an incidence rate of 4.4 per million [6].

Site Distribution

STSs may occur anywhere, but they are most commonly located in the thigh, buttock, groin (46%); trunk (18%); arm and knees (13%); pelvis (13%); and head and neck (9%) [7]. Most sarcomas of the extremities are deep-located and have a median diameter of 9 cm. It has been shown, on the other hand, that depth of the tumor constitute a sensitive marker of malignancy [8]. Retroperitoneal tumors become symptomatic only when reach a large size.

Etiology

The etiology of most STSs is not identified. In some cases, genetic, environmental and iatrogenic factors, viral infections and immune deficiency have been related to the development of malignant STS. Multistage cancerogenesis with progressive accumulation of genetic alterations accumulated in the cells and increasing histological malignancy have been hypothesized as a possible mechanism for pathogenesis of STS.

Genetic Factors

Li-Fraumeni syndrome, a familiar cancer syndrome resulting from a genetic loss of the tumor-suppressor gene p53, has been related to an increased incidence of STS and other malignancies. Neurofibromatosis (type 1) is characterized by multiple benign nerve tumors. In about 2% of cases benign nerve fibromas undergo malignant transformation to develop malignant peripheral nerve sheath tumors. Translocation t(X;18)(p11;q11), involving the nuclear transcription factor SYT and two breakpoints on chromosome X has been found in about 90% of synovial sarcomas. Furthermore, patients with translocations involving the second X breakpoint (SSX2) show a better outcome than those with translocations involving SSX1. Some types of STS such as desmoid tumors, multiple leyomiomas (often angiolipomas), neuroblastomas, and paragangliomas, have been reported to show a familial predisposition.

Environmental Factors

Several population based studies have associated exposure to chemical carcinogens including phenoxyacetic herbicides, chlorophenols and dioxin, with an increased incidence of STSs. Furthermore, a retrospective cohort study has evidenced a significantly higher mortality rate for STS in the cohort exposed to chemical carcinogens [9].

Iatrogenic Factors

Radiation induced STS is rare (<1%). Most cases have been associated with radiotherapy for breast cancer and lymphoma, being the risk directly related to dose (risk increases with a total radiation dose of 50 Gy or more), and the median time between exposure and tumor presentation of about 10 years. Some reports evidenced the development of malignant STS at fracture sites, in scar tissue, and close to surgical implants.

Viruses and Immunodeficiency

In immunodeficient patients, human herpes virus 8 have a key role in the pathogenesis of Kaposi sarcoma, while Epstein Barr virus has been related to the formation of smooth muscle tumors.

Classification

The complete WHO classification of soft tissue tumors is reported in Table 1. More than 50 different categories of STSs are distinguished on the basis of their histological appearances.

Leiomyosarcoma

In most series, the most common STS is leiomyosarcoma. The tumor occur more frequently in females than males (2:1), typically in the 5th and 6th decades of life. However, in rare cases, leiomyosarcoma can affect children [10]. This tumor derives from smooth muscle cells, most frequently in the uterus, gastrointestinal and urologic organs [11-13]. Leiomyosarcoma has classically been subdivided into three groups for prognostic and treatment purposes: leiomyosarcoma of somatic soft tissue, cutaneous leiomyosarcoma and leiomyosarcoma of vascular origin. The most common site of involvement of leiomyosarcoma is the retroperitoneum, accounting for approximately 50% of occurrences [14]. Since the 1970s there have been a number of cases of leiomyosarcoma reported in the setting of immune dysfunction (patients having undergone transplantation or treated with immunosuppressive therapies, or infected with the HIV virus) [15, 16]. Although these tumors are generally associated with small blood vessels, they usually do not present with signs or symptoms of vascular compression. However, given the fact that these tumors have increased access to blood vessels, the rate of metastatic spread is very high. Leiomyosarcoma, in fact, seems to be the most aggressive of all soft tissue tumors, in terms of metastasis and poor outcome [17, 18].

Malignant Fibrous Histiocytoma

In most series, the entity malignant fibrous histiocytoma (MHF) was previously identified as fibrosarcoma [19]. MHF is commonly localized in the lower extremities or trunk and usually originates in deep-seated skeletal muscles. These tumors appear as rapidly enlarging masses, painless and non-tender. They can present as superficial (dermal or subcutaneous) formations, which may reach only a few centimeters in diameter, or deep formations (retroperitoneum), which sometimes attain a diameter of 15 cm or greater. These tumors have a variety of histological patterns that were formerly considered to be distinct clinicopathologic entities. These lesions, which had been classified according to the basic cellular type, include fibroxanthoma, malignant fibroxanthoma, inflammatory fibrous histiocytoma, and giant cell tumor of soft part. Four histologic patterns are usually identified: storiform, mixoid, giant cell, and inflammatory. The storiform arrangement of tumor cells is characterized by fascicles of spindle cells that intersect to form a pinwheel pattern; abnormal giant and atypical cells may also be recognized. In the myxoid variant, the tumor cells are dispersed in a richly myxoid matrix. This variant has a better prognosis than the other patterns. The giant cell type is characterized by abundant osteoclast-like giant cells that are diffusely distributed among the malignant fibrohistiocytic elements. Occurrence of MHF has not been related to radiation exposure, bone infarction, implanted metallic or plastic devices [20, 21]. There are no estabilished laboratory or immunohistochemical markers to define outcome; recently, the presence of bone morphogenic protein-2 has been related to a better prognosis in patients with malignant fibrous histiocytoma [22].

Liposarcoma

Liposarcoma is the third most common STS in adults. The most common sites are the lower extremity and the abdomen (retroperitoneum). These tumors can attain great size, but are usually well circumscribed and mulitlobulated. Five histological subtypes can be distinguished: well-differentiated, myxoid, round cell, dedifferentiated, and pleomorphic. Well-differentiated liposarcomas are constituted by relatively mature fat and fibrocollagenous tissues, sometimes resembling lipomas. Inadequate sampling can therefore lead to a misdiagnosis of a benign lipoma. In rare cases, well-differentiated liposarcomas, usually after multiple local recurrences, transform into a high-grade spindle-cell sarcoma ("dedifferentiated liposarcoma"). This variant has a high risk of metastasize. The high-grade liposarcomas (round cell and pleomorphic) may disclose extensive hemorrhage and necrosis. Myxoid liposarcoma present as a plexiform capillary network associated with lipoblasts and mesenchimal cells. In round-cell liposarcomas, the lipoblasts are interspersed within poorly differentiated round cells. It has been supposed that the round cell and myxoid liposarcoma variants constitute the same malignant entity. This is supported by the discovery of a reciprocal translocation between chromosomes 12 and 16, which is common to both neoplasms. Pleomorphic liposarcoma presents a mixture of bizarre, multivacuolated, lipoblasts and atypical stromal cells, many of which contain abnormal mitotic figures. Unlike other soft-tissue sarcomas, liposarcomas may occur in multiple and unusual sites in the same individual. Therefore, careful physical inspection is recommended in a patient with a suspicious liposarcoma. High-grade liposarcomas should be treated as any other high-grade soft tissue sarcoma: neoadjuvant chemotherapy, wide surgical excision, and adjuvant chemotherapy. Radiation therapy is mandatory if wide margins were not achieved.

Fibrosarcoma

Fibrosarcoma was formerly considered the most common STS. However, histopathological features of the tumors varied considerably. Thus, after the term of "malignant fibrous histiocytoma" was assigned to the majority of these tumors, and particularly to the malignant one, fibrosarcoma has become uncommon. The diagnosis of fibrosarcoma is usually made by exclusion. The fundamental cell of this neoplasm is the fibroblast; atypical features and bizarre mitotic figures may be identified in the fibroblastic stroma. Fibrosarcoma usually arise in the upper and lower extremities, in the pelvis, and inside the bone [23]. Superficial variants are unusual. A typical t(12;15) translocation can be identified in children and young patients [24].

Synovial Sarcoma

Synovial sarcoma occurs in a younger age group than do most other sarcomas (average patient age<40). Lesions usually occur in joints, tendons, and ligaments, more frequently in the distal portion of the extremities. In spite of its name, there is no evidence to support the fact that this tumor arises directly from the synovial cells of a joint [25]. The synovial sarcoma typically appears as a deep-seated, well-circumscribed, firm, and multinodular mass. Unlike most STSs, synovial sarcomas may be dormant for years before becoming aggressive, and may be present as painless masses. A useful diagnostic sign may be evidenced by standard radiographs, that usually show small flecks of calcifications within the mass. Synovial sarcoma are high-grade tumors. Three histologic types can be distinguished: biphasic type, monophasic epithelial type, and monophasic fibrous type. The more common histological presentation of this tumor is a biphasic pattern. This is characterized by the presence of coexisting spindle cells and epithelioid cells. Within the spindle-cell population, areas resembling the branching vascular pattern of hemangiopericytoma may be identified. The epithelioid cell population sometimes includes gland-like structures. Immuno-histochemical stains of the glandular lamina show immunoreactivity for epithelial-type acid mucins and cytokeratine.

Rhabdomyosarcoma

Rhabdomyosarcomas were thought to arise from striated muscle, but there is little evidence for this [26]. Tumors are usually classified as embryonal (67%), alveolar (32%), and pleomorphic (1%), and they appear to occur more frequently in males than females (ratio 3:2) [6]. Alveolar and pleomorphic rhabdomyosarcomas are more common in adolescents, whereas embryonal type is more common in younger children. Pleomorphic and alveolar rabdhomyosarcoma commonly present with distant disease, in contrast to embryonal. A cytogenetic anomaly, described in chromosome 11p15.5, is now considered diagnostic; while some tumors show a trisomy 8 [27, 28]. Since the introduction of chemotherapy, most patients with childhood rabdhomyosarcoma survive [29].

Metastases

Differently from epithelial tumors, STSs metastasize mainly via hematogenic route. One tenth of the patients with high-grade STS have detectable metastases at presentation. Extremity sarcomas typically metastasize to the lungs in the early stages, and to the bones in later stages. Abdominal and pelvic sarcomas usually metastasize to the liver and lungs. Low-grade STSs have a very low metastatic potential (< 15%). STS involvement of regional lymph nodes is infrequent.

Diagnosis

Clinical Examination

Most STSs present as painless mass that has been growing for months. Tumors usually do not affect general health or limit functionality so may be accidentally discovered. Misinterpretation of these lesions as benign conditions may be common, given the rarity of STS and the apparently benign presentation. The most common anatomical localizations of STS are thigh, buttock, torso, upper extremities, retroperitoneum, and head and neck [30]. Current guidelines to simply identify a STS and to promptly refer patient to a specialized STSs centre are the soft tissue mass size and the depth of tumor

[31]. Superficial soft tissue masses larger than 5 cm and all deep-seated masses, irrespective of size, are more likely malignant [32].

Laboratory

Laboratory tests provides little information in relation to the STS.

Imaging

Ultrasound can be useful to rapidly distinguish between benign and suspicious lesions. Plain radiographs have a role in the evaluation of tumors that arise from bone. Synovial sarcoma and other STSs may show characteristic calcifications.

Magnetic Resonance imaging (MRI) is the gold standard imaging method for detecting, characterizing, and staging STS. The signal intensity of a tumor is assessed by comparing it with that of the adjacent muscle and fat. MRI provides the visualization of a lesion in all three planes (axial, sagittal, and coronal). MRI imaging is accurate in defining tumor size and relationships with muscle and fascial planes. Contrast-enhanced MRI also enables to define relationships of the tumor to the adjacent neurovascular structures. Most STSs are dark on T1 (hypo-intense) and light on T2 (hyper-intense). Masses with relatively high signal intensity on both T1 and T2 are lipoma, well-differentiated liposarcoma, haemangioma, subacute haemorrhage; while masses with low signal intensity on both T1 an T2 are desmoid or fibrosarcoma [33].

High resolution computed tomography (CT) is the gold standard for examining sarcomas of the abdomen and of the chest and for pre-operative staging. A baseline chest CT has a role in the early identification of bony involvement and for evidence of pulmonary metastases, especially for STS > 5 cm [34].

The role of positron emission tomography (PET) for diagnosis and monitoring of STS is still controversial. This technique is particularly indicated to detect the tumor biological activity; it can be used for differentiating benign lesions from malignant tumors, seeking metastases, additional masses, lymph nodes extensions, and evaluation of local recurrence and tumor response to chemotherapy [35].

Bone scan is currently used to determine the involvement of a bone by an adjacent STS or the tumor vascularization [36].

Biopsy

A histological diagnosis is an essential part of the workup and of the treatment protocol. Open incision biopsy has a relatively high complication rate (12-17%) but a great diagnostic accuracy [37]; in particular, it constitutes the ideal approach for extremity masses. Limb masses are usually sampled through a small longitudinal incision, considering that the whole mass will be definitely resected at the time of the surgical intervention. A sufficient amount of tissue is usually necessary to provide frozen and permanent sections for classification and grading of the tumor, for immunohistochemical detection of particular tumor markers such as p53, S-100, and cytokeratin [38, 39], for studies of DNA ploidy through flow cytometry assays [40], and for the study with the scanning electron microscope. Core needle biopsy is the standard approach for deep-seated lesions, it is a very safe procedure but sometimes not definitive and inaccurate. Various studies, however, showed that core needle biopsy has a diagnostic sensitivity of 90-95% [37, 41]. Excisional biopsy is not recommended, particularly for masses more than 2 cm in diameter, since such a procedure may contaminate surrounding tissues, making necessary a wider re-excision of the area. Fine needle aspiration cytology is rarely recommended in the early diagnostic phase of a suspicious lesion, given the limited amount of available sample, which affects not only diagnostic sensitivity but also the possibility to identify tumor lineage through methods such as cytogenetics and immunocytochemistry. It may find a role in confirming tumor recurrence [42].

Ultrasound, CT or MRI guided biopsies are used when the mass is difficult to identify or necrotic [43]. It is essential to have caution in the selection of an appropriate pathway, cooperation with the treating physician, and careful review of the biopsy tissue by a pathologist who is experienced in diagnosing sarcomas.

Lymph node biopsies are not usually indicated in patients with STS. Lymph node metastasis, in fact, occur only in 5% of cases, except in cases of synovial and epithelioid sarcoma, angiosarcoma, clear cell sarcoma (melanoma of the soft tissue) and rhabdomyosarcoma, where incidence of modal metastases may be evidenced in more than 10%. In these cases, therapeutic lymphadenectomy with curative aim has been related to a 5-year overall survival of 46% versus less than 1% in case of no lymphadenectomy or non-curative lymphadenectomy [44]. Another approach is constituted by first excising the tumor, and then, after the margin is determined to be negative on the histological revision, by scheduling a nuclear medicine radiotracer study to analyze the drainage of the tumor bed and to identify the sentinel lymph node (lymph node with the highest level of activity).

Staging and Grading

Two staging systems are currently used - the Musculoskeletal Tumor Society (MSTS) staging system and the American Joint Commission on Cancer staging system (GTNM). Both of these systems consider the tumor size and grade of malignancy. The GNTM (grading, tumor nodes, metastases) system is shown in Table 2.

Prognosis

The most important prognostic factors are the histological grade, tumor size, and relationship to fascial planes. Low-grade, small in size and confined tumors have a good prognosis and may be cured only with surgery; while high-grade, large in size, metastasizing or locally recurrent tumors usually require more aggressive treatments, such as adjunctive or neoadjunctive chemotherapy or radiotherapy [45, 46]. The median overall survival of patients with stage IV disease is 12 months.

Table 2. TNM staging system of soft tissue tumors

Primary tumor (T)	TX: primary tumor cannot be assessed
	T0: no evidence of primary tumor
	T1: tumor < 5 cm in greatest dimension
	T1a: superficial tumor
	T1b: deep tumor
	T2: tumor > 5 cm in greatest dimension
Regional lymph nodes (N)	NX: regional lymph nodes cannot be assessed
	N0: no regional lymph node metastasis
	N1: regional lymph node metastasis
Distant metastasis (M)	M0: no distant metastasis
	M1: distant metastasis
Histopathological Grading (G)	G1: well differentiated
	G2: Moderately differentiated
	G3: Poorly differentiated
	G4: Undifferentiated

Stage Grouping

Stage IA	T1a,b	N0	M0	G1,2
Stage IB	T2a	N0	M0	G1,2
Stage IIA	T2b	N0	M0	G1,2
Stage IIB	T1	N0	M0	G3,4
Stage IIC	T2a	N0	M0	G3,4
Stage III	T2b	N0	M0	G3,4
Stage IVA	Any T	N1	M0	Any G
Stage IVB	Any T	Any N	M1	Any G

Treatment

Appropriate management of STS requires cooperation of a multidisciplinary team of surgeons, pathologists, radiation oncologists and clinical oncologists [47]. Patients with suspect STS must be carefully studied with anamnestic investigation, clinical examination, laboratory tests, CT of the tumor site, x-ray or CT of the chest, MRI of the tumor site, bone scan, PET scan to evidence the distance metastases, and, finally, histological examination of the lesion. In all cases, the aim of multidisciplinary therapy is minimizing local and distance recurrence and preserving a functional limb and a good post-operative quality of life.

Surgery

Surgery is the principal treatment in patients with localized disease. Limb-sparing surgery is the standard surgical approach for most patients with STS of the upper and lower extremities [48]. A well-executed surgery should include a wide excision with a negative margin, incorporating the biopsy site. European guidelines considers 1 cm of normal tissue an acceptable resection margin [49]. Categories of surgical margins are classified as follows: 1) intralesional; 2) marginal; 3) wide; 4) radical. An intralesional surgery passes through the reactive margins of the tumor directly into the tumor cavity; surgical field remains potentially contaminated, and macroscopic tumor is left behind. A marginal excision is defined as a removal of the entire tumor without removing normal tissue; satellite tumor cells may remain in the reactive tissue. A wide intracompartmental *"en-bloc"* resection is the removal of entire tumor including at least 2 cm margin of adjacent normal tissue; the risk of a local recurrence is very low. A radical excision (extracompartmental) means the remotion of the entire bone/ muscle compartment, with a minimal risk of local recurrence [50]. Generally, surgery alone may be sufficient for any size low grade sarcoma, and for high grade sarcoma smaller than 5 cm.

Adjuvant radiotherapy may be helpful in reducing the risk of local recurrence or metastases. In particular, adjuvant radiotherapy should follow surgery when the excision margins is close, or there is extramuscular involvement.

Reconstructive surgery usually involves the use of muscle flaps or free flaps. Most resections will require durable tissue coverage, particularly if adjuvant radiation therapy is scheduled [51].

Hemorrhage, infections and deep venous thrombosis are some frequent complications of surgery.

Limb salvage approaches are not indicated when tumor is proximal to neurovascular structures so that tumor-free margins are not achievable, or when the risks of adjuvant radiotherapy are not affordable. Amputation may be considered when limb-sparing surgery is not indicated.

In patients with high stage disease, surgery may constitute a proper palliative therapy. In any case, surgeons should carefully discuss with the patient about the surgical morbidity and the post-operative rehabilitative process. Furthermore, functional post-operative rehabilitation should require an intensive interdisciplinary cooperation among nurses, physioterapists, and occupational therapists.

Adjuvant and Neoadjuvant Chemotherapy

For most STSs, the role of systemic chemotherapy is still controversial. Specifically, its value depends on the histological type of STS. Adjuvant chemotherapy is strongly indicated in the treatment of rhabdomyosarcoma and Ewing's sarcoma, because of the very high risk of metastatic spread [52]. Other histological types, such as synovial sarcoma and myxoid liposarcoma, are most likely chemosensitive. Several randomized trials showed a significant improvement in disease-free survival and loco-regional control in case of ifosfamide and doxorubicin-based chemotherapy [53-55]. The protocol MAID (mesna, doxorubicin, ifosfamide, dacarbazine) has shown a significant efficacy in high grade large extremities STS. The protocol is given pre-operatively for three courses; every cycle is followed by radiation therapy (22Gy), and surgery is performed at about three weeks after the end of the third cycle [56]. Common side effects of chemotherapy are gastrointestinal and hematological toxicity.

Chemotherapy may be administered in selected cases of advanced disease as a palliative approach.

Isolated Limb Perfusion

Isolated limb perfusion is a procedure based on intra-arterial or intravenous infusion of high concentration of melphalan and tumor necrosis factor to a limb isolated by tourniquet compression, under hyperthermic conditions. This technique can be used to reduce tumor size or for palliative intent. Several multicenter studies found a rate of limb salvage of about 85% for intermediate or high grade STSs treated with this procedure [57].

Radiotherapy

Radiation therapy is often used to reduce the risk of local recurrence and metastases [58, 59]. It may be pre-operatively, intra-operatively and post-operatively [58]. It is particularly indicated for intermediate or high grade STSs, large deep low grade STSs and tumors involving important anatomical structures (such as neurovascular structures) that cannot be completely resected [60]. The total radiation dose given to a patient ranges from 40 to 60 Gy or more, on the basis of the tumor localization, the extent of the surgery, and the presence of microscopical or macroscopical disease.

Brachytherapy (or interstitial therapy), where a radioactive source is implanted within the tumor bed after surgical resection for 3 days, has been showed to have the same efficacy than standard radiotherapy, and to be less expensive and time-sparing.

Treatment Of Metastatic Disease

Metastatic STSs are mainly incurable, but a few patients achieve a durable complete response, becoming long-term survivors. Some patients benefit from surgical resection of metastases. Doxorubicin and ifosfamide are drugs commonly used as first-line chemotherapy. Gemcitabine with or without docetaxel and dacarbazine have shown some activity in patients with leiomyosarcoma. Angiosarcoma partially respond to taxanes, while rhabdomyosarcoma and Ewing's sarcoma may benefit from vincristine, etoposide, and irinotecan administration.

Prognosis and Follow-up

Prognosis for STS depends on early diagnosis and control of local and distant disease. Most metastases from STS are to the lung and, less commonly, the lymph nodes. A recurrence of 9% has been showed in STS patients after a disease-free interval of five years [61]. Close follow-up is recommended, including careful physical examination to look for local recurrence. Ultrasound or MRI are recommended to investigate possible recurrences as well. Chest X-ray constitutes the exam of choice to detect pulmonary metastases; CT scan is the second choice for suspicious lesions [62]. For high grade tumors, recommendations of the European Society for Medical Oncology indicate to perform follow-up every 3-4 months in the first 3 years from diagnosis, every 6 months in the fourth-fifth years from diagnosis, and annually after five years from diagnosis. Low grade tumors require a frequency of follow-up of 4-6 months for the first five years, and annually after five years from diagnosis.

Bone Sarcomas

Primary tumors of the skeleton are rare. The highest incidence is found in children and adolescents, but their etiology is practically unknown. Bone metastases are the most frequent bone lesions in older patients. Signs and symptoms are often varied and diagnosis may be difficult, especially if conducted in non-specialized centers. Plan radiography and magnetic resonance imaging (MRI) are fundamental for the discovery and the primary characterization of bone lesions. The gold standard procedure for diagnosis is biopsy. Prevention and management of pathological fractures is recommended. Surgery, chemotherapy and radiotherapy should be performed after adequate disease staging.

Incidence

Bone sarcomas are very rare neoplasms; in 2009, approximately 2,570 new cases of cancer of the bones and joints were diagnosed in the United States.

Epidemiology

Osteosarcoma (OS) is the most frequent primary cancer of bone (excluding multiple myeloma). The annual incidence of osteosarcoma is approximately 0.2–0.03/100 000. The incidence is higher in adolescents (0.8–1.1/100 000/year at age 15–19), although peak have been noted in the elderly affected by Paget's disease and previous radiation therapy. Chondrosarcoma (CS) is one of the most frequent bone sarcomas of adulthood. The incidence is approximately 0.1/100 000 per year. Ewing's sarcoma (ES) is the third most common primary malignant bone cancer, mainly occurring in children and adolescents, at an incidence of 0.3/100 000 per year. Malignant fibrous histiocytoma (MFH) and fibrosarcoma represent only between 2% and 5% of primary bone malignancies, mainly occurring in adults. Other very rare bone sarcomas include specific entities such as angiosarcoma, liposarcoma, adamantinoma and chordoma. Males are more frequently affected than females. Parosteal sarcoma, a low-grade variant of osteosarcoma, is evidenced more frequently in females. OS has *no race-predilection*, whereas ES has *a strong predilection* for Caucasians [63].

Etiology

For the majority of bone sarcomas, our understanding of risk factors is very limited.

Genetic Factors
Li-Fraumeni syndrome is often associated with an increased risk of bone sarcomas, as well as other malignancies such as breast cancer, soft tissues sarcoma, brain and adrenal tumors, and leukemia. Germ-line deletion of the chromosome 13q14 in children with inherited retinoblastoma is associated with an increased incidence of bone sarcomas.

Environmental Factors
A traumatic event is sometimes involved. Preexisting benign tumors or other pathological conditions can be associated with the development of OS (Paget's disease, fibrous dysplasia). CS can arise from solitary or multiple hereditary exosostosis. MHF can develop from sites of bone infarct.

Iatrogenic Factors
Therapeutic irradiation can cause bone sarcomas. The tumor usually arises within the irradiated field after a "window" period of at least 3 years. Patients with the germline mutation in the 13q14 locus (retinoblastoma gene) have a significantly higher risk of developing post-irradiation OS.

OS has been also related to previous chemotherapy for unrelated malignancies (anthracyclines and alkylating drugs). Rare cases of bone sarcomas have been evidenced in the site of implantation of metallic orthopedic devices.

Classification

The WHO classification of bone sarcomas recognizes several histological subtypes (Table 3). The most common non-hematopoietic malignant tumors are OS, CS, ES, and MHF. The most common hematopoietic malignant tumors of bone are plasma cell tumors.

Osteosarcoma

OS is the most common primary bone sarcoma, accounting for about 45% of the total. It is a spindle cell tumor which typically produces osteoid or immature bone matrix. Most OSs occur during childhood and adolescence. When occurring in the third or fourth decade of life, OS is usually associated with a preexisting benign condition such as Paget's disease or with irradiated bone. The male-female ratio is 1.5 to 2. Between 80% and 90% of OS occur in the metaphysis of long bon; the most common sites are the distal femur, proximal tibia, and proximal humerus. Histologically, the tumor is characterized by a malignant stroma that produces an osteoid matrix.

The stroma is constituted by an arrangement of pleomorphic cells with hyperchromatic and irregular nuclei, and mitotic and atypical figures. OSs are usually classified on the basis of the predominant tissue type. The "osteoblastic" category include those tumors in which the predominant stromal type is the malignant osteoid. Calcification of the matrix can also be present. The "chondroblastic" variant is characterized by the production of malignant cartilage. Alternatively, the "fibroblastic" OS reveals large areas of proliferating fibroblasts arranged in intersecting fascicles. The "telangiectatic" variant consists of numerous blood-filled cystic and sinusoidal spaces of variable size. The most usual clinical sign is the presence of a tender, soft tissue swelling, accompanied by pain. Plain radiography evidences a destructive tumor with increased intramedullary radiodensity, a pattern of invasion of the surrounding bone, cortical destruction, periosteal reaction, extension to adjacent tissues, and soft-tissue calcification. The periosteum may

Table 3. WHO classification of bone tumors

CARTILAGE TUMOURS	HAEMATOPOIETIC TUMORS
Benign	Plasma cell myeloma
Osteochondroma	Malignant lymphoma, NOS
Chondroma	
Enchondroma	GIANT CELL TUMOR
Periosteal chondroma	Giant cell tumor
Multiple chondromatosis	Malignancy in giant cell tumor
Chondroblastoma	
Chondromyxoid fibroma	NOTOCHORDAL TUMORS
Chondrosarcoma	Chordoma
Central, primary, and secondary	
Peripheral	VASCULAR TUMORS
Dedifferentiated	Haemangioma
Mesenchymal	Angiosarcoma
Clear cell	
	SMOOTH MUSCLE TUMORS
OSTEOGENIC TUMORS	Leiomyoma
Osteoid osteoma	Leiomyosarcoma
Osteoblastoma	
Osteosarcoma	LIPOGENIC TUMORS
Conventional	Lipoma
chondroblastic	Liposarcoma
fibroblastic	
osteoblastic	NEURAL TUMORS
Telangiectatic	Neurilemmoma
Small cell	
Low grade central	MISCELLANEOUS TUMORS
Secondary	Adamantinoma
Parosteal	Metastatic malignancy
Periosteal	
High grade surface	MISCELLANEOUS LESIONS
	Aneurysmal bone cyst
FIBROGENIC TUMORS	Simple cyst
Desmoplastic fibroma	Fibrous dysplasia
Fibrosarcoma	Osteofibrous dysplasia
	Langerhans cell histiocytosis
FIBROHISTIOCYTIC TUMORS	Erdheim-Chester disease
Benign fibrous histiocytoma	Chest wall hamartoma
Malignant fibrous histiocytoma	
	JOINT LESIONS
EWING SARCOMA/PRIMITIVE	Synovial chondromatosis
NEUROECTODERMAL TUMOR	
Ewing sarcoma	

be elevated by a reactive new bone formation; this determines a distinctive radiologic feature called "Codman's triangle". Radiologically, OSs can be classified into three groups: sclerotic osteosarcomas (30%), osteolytic osteosarcomas (25%), and mixed pattern (45%). OS must be differentiate from giant-cell tumor, aneurysmal bone cyst, fibrosarcoma, and MFH of bone. The standard schedule for management of OS is constituted by preoperative chemotherapy followed by limb-sparing surgery, followed by post-operative chemotherapy. Most OSs are radioresistant.

Chondrosarcoma

CS is the second most common primary bone sarcoma, constituting about 20-25% of all bone sarcomas. It usually occurs in adulthood or old age (peak incidence between the ages of 40 and 60). The preferential sites are the pelvis, femur, and shoulder girdle. The basis malignant tissue is cartilaginous, with no evidence of primary osteoid formation. The histological classification includes enchondroma, osteochondroma, chondroblastoma, chondromyxofibroma, periosteal chondroma, and synovial chondromatosis. A further classification divides central CSs, that arise from within the medullary canal, and peripheral CSs, that arise from the surface of the bone. CSs are histologically graded as I (low), II (intermediate), or III (high); the majority are grade I or II. CSs usually present with pain. Pelvic CSs commonly present with referred pain to the lower back, sciatic pain, urinary obstruction, unilateral swelling of the lower extremity due to iliac vein obstruction, or a painless pelvic mass. On standard radiographs, central lesions appear as well-defined lytic formations with punctate calcification. Diagnoses can be relatively easy for high-grade tumors; sometimes it may be difficult to distinguish low-grade CS from other benign cartilage tumors. In the latter case, correlation of the clinical, radiographic, and histological data becomes essential for accurate diagnosis. The prognosis and therapy of primary and central secondary CSs are the same. Surgery is the preferred treatment for all CSs, while the use of neoadjuvant and adjuvant chemotherapy is not well estabilished. Low- and intermediate-grade CSs are resistant to chemotherapy. Chemotherapy, however, should be administered to any young patient with a high-grade tumor. Post-operative radiotherapy is always recommended.

Ewing's sarcoma

ES constitutes 10 to 15% of all bone sarcoma and is the third most common bone sarcoma. It preferentially occurs in the White population; while it is very rare to diagnose ES in a Black patient. The peak incidence is the second decade of life. It usually involves the long bones and the flat bones of skeletally immature patients. The tumor mass is usually composed of small, undifferentiated, round, blue mesenchymal cells that are rich in glycogen (periodic acid-Shiff positive cells). The small round cells grow in solid, densely packed sheets and nests. They have round, centrally located nuclei with indistinct cytoplasmic features. Often a biphasic pattern can be revealed by the presence of "light" and "dark" cells (i.e., cells with an open chromatin structure and cells with dark condensed nuclei, respectively). The "dark" cells constitute apoptotic tumor cells. Common differential diagnoses are metastatic neuroblastoma, large-cell lymphoma (in the young age group), acute leukemia (in the young age group) and small-cell carcinoma (in patients older than 30). A typical karyotypic marker for ES is a reciprocal chromosomal translocation, t(11;22)(q24;q12) that results in a chimeric protein, EWS/FLI-1. This translocation occurs in approximately 90% of ES. On standard radiography, ES appears as a destructive intramedullary lesion that affects the diaphysis. These tumors usually produce a diffuse and irregular periosteal reaction ("onion-skin appearance"), as well as a wide spread through the cortex and soft-tissue components. ES is an extremely malignant tumor with high rates of metastatic disease and local recurrence following surgery alone. The most common sites of metastases are lung, bones, and bone marrow. Given the use of new multimodality treatments that include combinations of chemotherapy, surgery, and radiation therapy, the 5-year survival rate has dramatically increased, being around 80% with effective therapy.

Metastases

A large majority of patients with high-grade primary bone sarcomas have distant micro metastasis at diagnosis. The most common site of distant metastases is the lungs. Other usual sites are bones, bone marrow, and viscera. For this reason, the best standard of cure for high-grade bone sarcoma is constituted by combination of surgery and systemic chemotherapy. Regional node involvement is rare.

Clinical Presentation

Sarcomas may involve any bone. Most OSs arises in the metaphysis of a long bone. About 50% of ESs arises in the extremities, while 25% involves the pelvic bones, and 25% the ribs and the vertebral column. Sacral and spine involvement is very rare. The clinical presentation of patients with bone tissue sarcoma is not specific, so that a long time interval may pass until the tumor is identified.

Local Symptoms

Localized pain, swelling and limited mobility are the main distinctive symptoms of bone sarcomas. Spontaneous fracture may also be present as a sign. Although the pain may initially be mild and transient, it might finally become more severe and unremitting, occurring during night and spreading into the adjacent join. In severe cases, pain may need opioid therapy. Pressure on the nerve roots can cause burning or radiating pain.

Patients often present with a mass, typically rapidly increasing in size. Swelling may be accompanied by skin changes such as warmth, erythema, tensed skin, marked veins, striation and ulceration. Usually, malignant masses cannot not be freely mobile.

Limitation of movement can occur in case of direct involvement of the joint (especially in OS and CS), or in case of secondary synovitis in the joint.

Pathological fracture may occur early in cases of benign lesions, while it is a rather late event in case of malignant tumors.

Constitutional Symptoms

General symptoms are rare in patients with bone sarcoma. Symptoms such as fever, malaise, and loss of weight may occur in patients with ES [64].

Diagnosis

Physical Examination

Clinical examination should be performed to establish tumor size, the mobility of the mass respect to skin, subcutis and musculature, and eventual skin changes.

Laboratory

No specific laboratory abnormalities are evidenced in patients with bone tumors. Increased levels of serum lactic dehydrogenase, gamma glutamyltransferase, and erythrocyte sedimentation rate, might have a prognostic value in patients with ES [65, 66]. Serum alkaline phosphatase level has been recently considered a biologic marker of tumor activity in patients with OS, as well as a prognostic marker following neoadjuvant and adjuvant chemotherapy [65].

Imaging

Conventional X-ray is the first diagnostic tool for the characterization of osseous lesions and the differential diagnosis between benign and malignant tumors. Age is useful to hypothesize diagnosis: before 5 years of age, a malignant lesion is most commonly metastatic neuroblastoma; after 5 years, primary OS or ES; after 40 years, metastasis or myeloma. Important information to search in biplanar radiographs include tumor site, tumor extent, the presence and the extent of bone destruction, the pattern of periosteal reaction, and the type of matrix within the tumor. Some tumors are more common in particular bones. For example, the most common sites for adamantinoma in adults are tibia and fibula, while the most usual localization for chondroblastoma in children is epiphysis of long bones. The evaluation of the tumor size is an important part of diagnosis and staging. A tumor less than 6 cm in maximum diameter is probably benign, while one more than 6 cm is considered potentially malignant. There are three different patterns of bone destruction which indicate a variable aggressiveness of the tumor. The geographic pattern is the least aggressive pattern of bone destruction, as it is characteristic of a slow-growing tumor. The tumor may or may not be surrounded by a sclerotic rim; in both cases the margins of the lesion are very well defined and distinct from the surrounding normal bone. A lesion with geographic pattern that has no sclerosis and has a cortical limit expanded more than 1 cm beyond the original cortical shape, is defined as moderately aggressive. The moth-eaten pattern is characterized by multiple medium-sized holes randomly distributed in the bone; it is indicative of a lesion with a more aggressive growth. The permeative pattern indicates a very aggressive bone tumor. The lesion is indistinct from the surrounding normal bone. Periosteal reaction indicates the tumor-induced new bone formation associated with erosion of the cortex. The presence of periosteal reaction depends upon the rate of aggressiveness of the tumor. Most tumors appear radiolucent, suggesting that they have no matrix or the matrix is not mineralized. Some lesions, such as cartilaginous tumors, produce matrix that calcifies or ossifies.

Standard CT should be used in the case of a diagnostic doubt. CT provides better assessment of calcification, ossification, periosteal reaction, reactive sclerosis, and soft tissue involvement than standard radiography. Abdominal and chest CT are particular important tools in the staging process. CT is critical for evaluation of pulmonary nodules, masses, and lymphadenopathy.

MRI is the examination of choice in the evaluation of the relationship of the tumor to the soft-tissue, to the neurovascular structures or to the joint. MRI is also the preferred modality to evaluate the intramedullary extent of the tumor, as well as the presence of skip metastases within the bone. Furthermore, MRI is the most sensitive imaging tool for diagnosing local recurrences of bone sarcomas.

PET is useful for detection of local recurrence, metastatic disease, as well as for evaluation of response to treatment.

Biopsy

Biopsy is gold standard for diagnosis. It should be carried out by a surgeon or a radiologist expert in percutaneous biopsy techniques at a reference center. Tissue may be obtained by core needle biopsy (multiple) or open biopsy. Biopsy should guarantee a minimal contamination of normal tissue. To be sure that the biopsy location is adequate, it is recommended to operate under ultrasound guidance, or to perform X-ray or CT prior to procedure.

Table 4. TNM staging system of bone tumors

Primary tumor (T)	TX: primary tumor cannot be assessed T0: no evidence of primary tumor T1: tumor < 8 cm in greatest dimension T2: tumor > 8 cm in greatest dimension T3: discontinuous tumors in the primary bone site
Regional lymph nodes (N)	NX: regional lymph nodes cannot be assessed N0: no regional lymph node metastasis N1: regional lymph node metastasis
Distant metastasis (M)	MX: distant metastasis cannot be assessed M0: no distant metastasis M1: distant metastasis M1a: lung M1b: other distant sites
Histopathological Grading (G)	GX: grade cannot be assessed G1: well differentiated-low grade G2: Moderately differentiated-low grade G3: Poorly differentiated-high grade G4: Undifferentiated-high grade (Ewing sarcoma is always classified as G4)

Staging and Grading

The MSTS (Musculoskeletal Tumor Society) staging system is currently used for the staging of bone sarcomas (Table 4). It is based on grade and tumor extent. Stage I is low grade, stage II is high grade, and stage III indicates the presence of distant metastases, independently from the extent of local tumor. Tumors A have only intra osseous involvement, while tumors B have extra osseous extent.

Stage Grouping

Stage IA	T1	N0	M0	G1,2 low grade
Stage IB	T2	N0	M0	G1,2 low grade
Stage IIA	T1	N0	M0	G3,4 high grade
Stage IIB	T2	N0	M0	G3,4 high grade
Stage III	T3	N0	M0	Any G
Stage IVA	Any T	N0	M1a	Any G
Stage IVB	Any T	N1	Any M	Any G
	Any T	Any N	M1b	Any G

Prognosis

Generally, primary bone cancers tend to be aggressive with fair to good cure rates. The most important factor in determining the prognosis of bone sarcoma is the presence of metastasis at diagnosis. Other prognostic variables related to moderate to good outlook are the tumor size (low volume) and anatomic site (peripheral) in patients with OS and ES. Furthermore, tumor response to adjuvant chemotherapy is an important prognostic factor for localized, operable extremity OS [67]. For OS and MFH, survival rates improve if age more than 10 years, distal extremity disease, good initial responsiveness to preoperative chemotherapy, small tumor size. Most CS tend to have low grade of malignancy and thus have a higher survival rate. Common 11;22 translocation, generating EWS-FLI1 fusion, has a positive prognostic value in ES [68]. For cases of localized bone cancer, the current overall five-year survival rate is about 55%-70% for OS patients, 70% for ES patients, 80% for CS patients, and 60% for patients with spindle cell sarcoma. For cases of metastatic bone cancer, OS and ES overall survival is approximately 30%; CS overall survival is between 10-30%, while spindle cell sarcoma overall survival is about 25% at five years from diagnosis.

Treatment

Surgery

Patients with sarcoma often require a combination of surgery, chemotherapy, and radiation therapy. Surgical excision is the standard treatment for bone sarcoma. It should be performed only after adequate pre-operative staging and, eventually, neo-adjuvant chemotherapy. Limb-sparing techniques were developed in the early 1970 [69]. Various types of resection are recognized, basing on the anatomic localization and the extent of the tumor to be excised: 1) intralesional; 2) marginal; 3) wide; 4) radical. After tumor resection, the following surgical phases include skeletal reconstruction and soft-tissue coverage.

Large skeletal and osteoarticular defects are mostly reconstructed by prosthetic arthroplasty. Alternative procedures of reconstruction are osteoarticular allografts or composite allografts (constituted by allograft placed over a protesis), vascular allo and autografts.

Soft tissue coverage should be extremely adequate to guarantee the success of the limb-salvage procedure. Regional muscle transfer is a useful technique to provide a vascularized flap, to reduce the infective risk, and to favorite a return of movement.

Contraindications to limb-sparing surgery are a major neurovascular involvement, as it makes unlikely a successful resection, and the presence of pathological fractures, which could favorite the tumor diffusion into the systemic circulation.

Currently, 80% to 85% of patients with primary malignant bone tumors involving the extremities can be treated prudently with conservative surgery. On the other hand, amputation still constitutes a standard therapeutic approach in patients in whom a limb-sparing procedure is not recommended.

Large growing tumors that are poor responders to chemotherapy and tumors infiltrating the skin, nerves and arteries, are often best managed by amputation [70].J Bone Joint Surg Am 1986;68:1331 Furthermore, amputations tend to be more frequent in very young children. In these patients, in fact, the limb length discrepancy after limb-sparing surgery would be disproportionate. The primary objectives of any oncologic therapy are effective local tumor control, decreased incidence of recurrence, and improved overall survival. In comparing limb-sparing procedures with amputation, local recurrence associated with limb-sparing resection is slightly higher than it is after amputation, but this has not been shown to reduce overall survival [71, 72].

Chemotherapy

Before routine use of systemic chemotherapy for the therapy of malignant sarcomas, overall survival was fewer than 20% at 5 years. Moreover, pulmonary metastasis occurred in 50% of patients, within 6 months of surgical resection. It was demonstrated that most patients had microscopical metastases at the time of diagnosis [73]. Several clinical studies showed that treatment with chemotherapy before surgery can increase overall survival in patients with OS. Common treatment programs include doxorubicin, cisplatin, high-dose methotrexate (followed by leucovorin rescue), and ifosfamide. Cycles are commonly given over periods of 6-12 months. Chemotherapy should be given also to older patients with OS using appropriate reduced-intensity protocols. Systemic therapy for ES consist of doxorubicin, cyclophosphamide, ifosfamide, vincristine, dactinomycin and etoposide. All current protocols employ four-to-six drug combinations of these substances. Usually, the sequencing schedule is neoadjuvant chemotherapy, followed by surgery and radiotherapy, and adjuvant chemotherapy. Treatment duration is about 10-12 months. High-dose chemotherapy followed by autologous stem cell transplantation is still under investigation in patients affected by poor-risk and metastatic ES. Adult patients should be treated with the same approach, taking into account the fact that tolerability of therapy might be low in this subgroup of patients.

Chemotherapy treatment can result in multiorgan dysfunction, and patients undergoing these therapies must be strictly observed and receive adequate supportive care in reference institutions. Sperm banking is recommended for male patients of reproductive age; female patients should consult a fertility physician.

Radiation Therapy

The role of adjuvant radiation therapy for OS is not well established. Patients with positive surgical margins and poor response to chemotherapy have a high risk of local recurrence. Doses in the range of 60 Gy are typically utilized. Patients with ES are usually treated with chemotherapy and radiation therapy. The schedule usually includes 45 Gy to the pre-chemotherapy mass plus a 2-cm margin, followed by a 10.8 Gy boost to the residual volume after chemotherapy. Intensity-modulated radiotherapy and proton therapy are alternative methods of treatment to be considered in OS. Proton beam radiotherapy can achieve a good local control in CS. ES is a radiation-responsive tumor. Combination of chemotherapy and radiotherapy can achieve local control of disease. Moreover, a dose of 45 Gy is recommended when incomplete surgery has occurred (microscopic or gross positive margins remain after resection).

Treatment of Metastatic Disease

The most usual site of metastatic spread for OS is the lungs. The surgical removal of all metastatic foci is recommended, usually by exploratory thoracotomy. Approximately 30% to 40% of patients who develop resectable lung metastases become long-term survivors. These patients may also benefit from aggressive reinduction chemotherapy. Patients with recurrent OS may benefit from new chemotherapeutic combinations, such as combination of cyclophosphamide and topotecan, or gemcitabine and docetaxel. Patients with unresectable lung metastases or extrapulmonary metastasis have a very poor prognosis; approximately 10% of such patients may become long-term survivors.

Aggressive combination chemotherapy (ifosfamide plus etoposide) and radiation therapy may lead to progression-free survival in patients with metastatic ES. Several promising non-randomized trials have investigating the role of intensive chemotherapy followed by autologous stem cell rescue, but the real efficacy is still unknown. Patients with lung metastases at diagnosis should be treated with consolidative low-dose, whole-lung irradiation following chemotherapy. The role of surgical resection of metastases in not well defined. Patients with painful bone metastases may benefit from palliative radiotherapy for pain control.

References

[1] Rydholm, A. Improving the management of soft tissue sarcoma. Diagnosis and treatment should be given in specialist centres. *BMJ,* 1998 317(7151), 93-4.

[2] Greenlee, RT; Murray, T; et al. Cancer statistics, 2000. *CA Cancer J. Clin.,* 2000 50(1), 7-33.

[3] Fleming, ID; Cooper, JS; et al. American Joint Committee on Cancer: Soft tissues. In: *AJCC Cancer Staging Manual,* Edition 5. Philadelphia: Lippincott-Raven; 1997:149–56.

[4] Gurney, JG; Young JL; et al. Soft tissue sarcomas (online). Available from: URL: http://seer.cancer.gov/publications/childhood/softtissue.pdf.

[5] Toro, JR; Travis, LB; et al. Incidence patterns of soft tissue sarcomas, regardless of primary site, in the surveillance, epidemiology and end results program, 1978-2001: An analysis of 26,758 cases. *Int. J. Cancer,* 2006 119(12), 2922-30.

[6] Perez, EA; Kassira, N; et al. Rhabdomyosarcoma in Children: A SEER Population Based Study. *J. Surg. Res.,* 2011 Mar 29. [Epub ahead of print].

[7] Lawrence, W Jr; Donegan, WL; et al. Adult soft tissue sarcomas. A pattern of care survey of the American College of Surgeons. *Ann. Surg,* 1987 205(4), 349-59.

[8] Hussein R, Smith MA. Soft tissue sarcomas: are current referral guidelines sufficient? *Ann. R. Coll. Surg. Engl,* 2005 87(3), 171-3.

[9] Kogevinas, M; Becher, H; et al. Cancer mortality in workers exposed to phenoxy herbicides, chlorophenols, and dioxins. An expanded and updated international cohort study. *Am. J. Epidemiol.,* 1997 145(12), 1061-75.

[10] De Saint Aubain Somerhausen, N; Fletcher, C. Leiomyosarcoma of Soft Tissue in Children: Clinicopathologic analysis of 20 cases. *Am. J. Surg. Pathol.,* 1999 23(7), 755.

[11] Friedrich, M; Villena-Heinsen ,C; et al. Leiomyosarcomas of the female genital tract: a clinical and histopathological study. *Eur. J. Gynaecol. Oncol.,* 1998 19(5), 470-5.

[12] Gallup, DG; Cordray, DR. Leiomyosarcoma of the uterus: case reports and a review. *Obstet. Gynecol. Surv.,* 1979 34(4), 300-12.

[13] Wang, HS; Chen, WS; et al. Leiomyosarcoma of the rectum: a series of twelve cases. *Zhonghua Yi Xue Za Zhi (Taipei),* 1996 57(4), 280-3.

[14] Golden, T; Stout, AP. Smooth muscle tumors of the gastrointestinal tract and retroperitoneal tissues. *Surg. Gynecol. Obstet.,* 1941 73, 784.

[15] Walker, D; Gill, TJ III; et al. Leiomyosarcoma in a renal allograft recipient treated with immunosuppressive drugs. *JAMA,* 1971 215, 2084.

[16] Ross, JS; Del Rosario, A; et al. Primary hepatic leiomyosarcoma in a child with the acquired immunodeficiency syndrome. *Hum. Pathol.,* 1992 23, 69.

[17] Gustafson, P; Willen, H; et al. Soft tissue leiomyosarcoma. A population-based epidemiologic and prognostic study of 48 patients, including cellular DNA content. *Cancer,* 1992 70(1), 114-9.

[18] Mankin, HJ; Casas-Ganem, J; et al. Leiomyosarcoma of somatic soft tissues. *Clin. Orthop. Relat. Res.,* 2004 421, 225-31.

[19] Fletcher, CD. Pleomorphic malignant fibrous histiocytoma: fact or fiction? A critical reappfaisal based on 159 tumors diagnosed as pleomorphic sarcoma. *Am. J. Surg. Pathol.*, 1992 16, 213-228.

[20] Keel, SB; Jaffe, KA; et al. Orthopaedic implant-related sarcoma: a study of twelve cases. *Mod. Pathol.,* 2001 14(10), 969-77.

[21] Lucas, DR; Miller, PR; et al. Arthroplasty-associated malignant fibrous histiocytoma: two case reports. *Histopathology*, 2001 39(6), 620-8.

[22] Asano, N; Yamakazi, T; et al. The expression and prognostic significance of bone morphogenetic protein-2 in patients with malignant fibrous histiocytoma. *J. Bone Joint Surg. Br.*, 2004 86(4), 607-12.

[23] Chow, LT; Lui, YH; et al. Primary sclerosing epithelioid fibrosarcoma of the sacrum: a case report and review of the literature. *J. Clin. Pathol.,* 2004 57(1), 90-4.

[24] Ferguson, WS. Advances in the adjuvant treatment of infantile fibrosarcoma. *Expert Rev. Anticancer The*r., 2003 3(2), 185-91.

[25] Miettinen, M; Virtanen, I. Synovial sarcoma--a misnomer. *Am. J. Pathol.,* 1984 117(1), 18-25.

[26] Pappo, AS; Shapiro, DN; et al. Biology and therapy of pediatric rhabdomyosarcoma. *J. Clin. Oncol.*, 1995 13(8), 2123-39.

[27] Kodet, R; Newton, WA Jr; et al. Rhabdoid tumors of soft tissues: a clinicopathologic study of 26 cases enrolled on the Intergroup Rhabdomyosarcoma Study. *Hum. Pathol.,* 1991 22(7), 674-84.

[28] Kilpatrick, SE; Teot, LA. Relationship of DNA ploidy to histology and prognosis in rhabdomyosarcoma. Comparison of flow cytometry and image analysis. *Cancer,* 1994 74(12), 3227-33.

[29] Raney, RB; Anderson, JR; et al. Rhabdomyosarcoma and undifferentiated sarcoma in the first two decades of life: a selective review of intergroup rhabdomyosarcoma study group experience and rationale for Intergroup Rhabdomyosarcoma Study V. *J. Pediatr. Hematol. Oncol.,* 2001 23(4), 215-20.

[30] Lawrence, W Jr; Donegan, WL; et al. Adult soft tissue sarcomas. A pattern of care survey of the American College of Surgeons. *Ann. Surg.,* 1987 205(4), 349-59.

[31] Hussein, R; Smith, MA. Soft tissue sarcomas: are current referral guidelines sufficient? *Ann. R. Coll. Surg. Engl.,* 2005 87(3), 171-3.

[32] Arca, MJ; Sondak, VK; et al. Diagnostic procedures and pretreatment evaluation of soft tissue sarcomas. *Semin. Surg. Oncol.,* 1994 10(5), 323-31.

[33] Kransdorf, MJ; Jelinek, JS; et al. Soft-tissue masses: diagnosis using MR imaging. *AJR Am. J. Roentgenol.*, 1989 153(3), 541-7.
[34] Grimer, R; Judson, I; et al. Guidelines for the management of soft tissue sarcomas. *Sarcoma,* 2010; 2010:506182. Epub 2010 May 31.
[35] Israel-Mardirosian, N; Adler, LP. Positron emission tomography of soft tissue sarcomas. Curr Opin Oncol, 2003 15(4), 327-30.
[36] Ilaslan, H; Schils, J; et al. Clinical presentation and imaging of bone and soft-tissue sarcomas. *Cleve Clin. J. Med.*, 2010 77, Suppl 1:S2-7.
[37] Strauss, DC; Qureshi, YA; et al. The role of core needle biopsy in the diagnosis of suspected soft tissue tumours. *J. Surg. Oncol.*, 2010 102(5), 523-9.
[38] Folpe, AL; Chand, EM; et al. Expression of Fli-1, a nuclear transcription factor, distinguishes vascular neoplasms from potential mimics. *Am. J. Surg. Pathol.,* 2001 25(8), 1061-6.
[39] Yoshikawa, H; Rettig, WJ; et al. Immunohistochemical detection of bone morphogenetic proteins in bone and soft-tissue sarcomas. *Cancer,* 1994 74(3), 842-7.
[40] Kilpatrick, SE; Teot, LA; et al. Relationship of DNA ploidy to histology and prognosis in rhabdomyosarcoma. Comparison of flow cytometry and image analysis. *Cancer,* 1994 74(12), 3227-33.
[41] De Marchi, A; Brach del Prever, EM; et al. Accuracy of core-needle biopsy after contrast-enhanced ultrasound in soft-tissue tumours. *Eur. Radiol.,* 2010 20(11), 2740-8.
[42] Rougraff, BT; Aboulafia, A; et al. Biopsy of soft tissue masses: evidence-based medicine for the musculoskeletal tumor society. *Clin. Orthop. Relat. Res.,* 2009 467(11), 2783-91.
[43] Hau, A; Kim, I; et al. Accuracy of CT-guided biopsies in 359 patients with musculoskeletal lesions. *Skeletal. Radiol.*, 2002 31(6), 349-53.
[44] Fong, Y; Coit, DG; et al. Lymph node metastasis from soft tissue sarcoma in adults. Analysis of data from a prospective database of 1772 sarcoma patients. *Ann. Surg.*, 1993 217(1), 72-7.
[45] Karakousis, CP; Emrich, LJ; et al. Soft-tissue sarcomas of the proximal lower extremity. *Arch. Surg.,* 1989 124(11), 1297-300.
[46] Simon, MA; Nachman, J. The clinical utility of preoperative therapy for sarcomas. *J. Bone Joint Surg. Am.*, 1986 68(9), 1458-63.
[47] Issels, RD; Schlemmer, M. Current trials and new aspects in soft tissue sarcoma of adults. *Cancer Chemother. Pharmacol.*, 2002 49 Suppl 1, S4-8.

[48] Misra, A; Mistry, N; et al. The management of soft tissue sarcoma. *J. Plast. Reconstr. Aesthet. Surg.*, 2009 62(2), 161-74.
[49] Grimer, R; Athanasou, N; et al. UK Guidelines for the Management of Bone Sarcomas. *Sarcoma* 2010 2010, 317462.
[50] Enneking, WF; Spanier, SS; et al. A system for the surgical staging of musculoskeletal sarcoma. 1980. *Clin. Orthop. Relat. Res.*, 2003 415, 4-18.
[51] Morii, T; Mochizuki, K; et al. Soft tissue reconstruction using vascularized tissue transplantation following resection of musculoskeletal sarcoma: evaluation of oncologic and functional outcomes in 55 cases. *Ann. Plast. Surg.*, 2009 62(3), 252-7.
[52] Heyn, R; Beltangady, M; et al. Results of intensive therapy in children with localized alveolar extremity rhabdomyosarcoma: a report from the Intergroup Rhabdomyosarcoma Study. *J. Clin. Oncol.*, 1989 7(2), 200-7.
[53] Rosenberg, SA; Kent, H; et al. Prospective randomized evaluation of the role of limb-sparing surgery, radiation therapy, and adjuvant chemoimmunotherapy in the treatment of adult soft-tissue sarcomas. *Surgery,* 1978 84(1), 62-9.
[54] Rosenberg, SA; Tepper, J; et al. Prospective randomized evaluation of adjuvant chemotherapy in adults with soft tissue sarcomas of the extremities. *Cancer,* 1983 52(3), 424-34.
[55] Scaife, CL; Pisters, PW. Combined-modality treatment of localized soft tissue sarcomas of the extremities. *Surg. Oncol. Clin. N. Am.,* 2003 12(2), 355-68.
[56] DeLaney, TF; Spiro, IJ; et al. Neoadjuvant chemotherapy and radiotherapy for large extremity soft-tissue sarcomas. *Int. J. Radiat. Oncol. Biol. Phys.*, 2003 56(4), 1117-27.
[57] Wray, CJ; Benjamin, RS; et al. Isolated limb perfusion for unresectable extremity sarcoma: Results of 2 single-institution phase 2 trials. *Cancer,* 2011 Jan 18. [Epub ahead of print].
[58] Suit, HD; Spiro, I. Role of radiation in the management of adult patients with sarcoma of soft tissue. *Semin. Surg. Oncol.*, 1994 10(5), 347-56.
[59] Levine, EA; Trippon, M; et al. Preoperative multimodality treatment for soft tissue sarcomas. *Cancer,* 1993 71(11), 3685-9.
[60] Casali, PG; Blay, JY. Soft tissue sarcomas: ESMO Clinical Practice Guidelines for diagnosis, treatment and follow-up. *Ann. Oncol.*, 2010 21 Suppl 5, v198-203.

[61] Stojadinovic, A; Leung, DH; et al. Primary adult soft tissue sarcoma: time-dependent influence of prognostic variables. *J. Clin. Oncol.*, 2002 20(21), 4344-52.
[62] Gortzak, E; Azzarelli, A; et al. A randomised phase II study on neo-adjuvant chemotherapy for 'high-risk' adult soft-tissue sarcoma. *Eur. J. Cancer,* 2001 37(9), 1096-103.
[63] Hogendoorn, PC; Athanasou, N; et al. Bone sarcomas: ESMO Clinical Practice Guidelines for diagnosis, treatment and follow-up. *Ann. Oncol,* 2010 21 Suppl 5, v204-13.
[64] Kissane, JM; Askin, FB; et al. Ewing's sarcoma of bone: clinicopathologic aspects of 303 cases from the Intergroup Ewing's Sarcoma Study. *Hum. Pathol.*, 1983 14(9), 773-9.
[65] Bacci, G; Ferrari, S; et al. Prognostic significance of serum LDH in Ewing's sarcoma of bone. *Oncol. Rep.*, 1999 6(4), 807-11.
[66] Hannisdal, E; Solheim, OP; et al. Alterations of blood analyses at relapse of osteosarcoma and Ewing's sarcoma. *Acta Oncol.*, 1990 29(5), 585-7.
[67] Merimsky, O; Kollender, Y; et al. Induction chemotherapy for bone sarcoma in adults: correlation of results with erbB-4 expression. *Oncol. Rep,* 2003 10(5), 1593-9.
[68] Lessnick, SL; Dacwag, CS; et al. The Ewing's sarcoma oncoprotein EWS/FLI induces a p53-dependent growth arrest in primary human fibroblasts. *Cancer Cell*, 2002 1(4), 393-401.
[69] Rosenberg, SA; Tepper, J; et al. The treatment of soft-tissue sarcomas of the extremities: prospective randomized evaluations of (1) limb-sparing surgery plus radiation therapy compared with amputation and (2) the role of adjuvant chemotherapy. *Ann. Surg,* 1982 196(3), 305-15.
[70] Harris, IE; Leff, AR; et al. Function after amputation, arthrodesis, or arthroplasty for tumors about the knee. *J. Bone Joint Surg. Am.*, 1990 72(10), 1477-85.
[71] Sluga, M; Windhager, R; et al. Local and systemic control after ablative and limb sparing surgery in patients with osteosarcoma. *Clin. Orthop. Relat. Res.,* 1999 (358),120-7.
[72] Rougraff, BT; Simon, MA; et al. Limb salvage compared with amputation for osteosarcoma of the distal end of the femur. A long-term oncological, functional, and quality-of-life study. *J. Bone Joint Surg. Am.*, 1994 76(5), 649-56.
[73] Bruland, OS; Høifødt, H; et al. Hematogenous micrometastases in osteosarcoma patients. *Clin. Cancer Res.*, 2005 11(13), 4666-73.

In: Sarcoma
Editor: Eric J. Butler

ISBN: 978-1-62100-362-5
© 2012 Nova Science Publishers, Inc.

Chapter II

Clinic-Histopathologic Diagnosis of the Kaposi's Sarcoma

Roberto Gabriel Albin[1]*
and Juan Carlos Perez-Cárdenas[2]**

[1]Internal Medicine Department "Freyre de Andrade" General Hospital, Habana Vieja, Havana City, Cuba
[2]Clinical Pathology Department "Freyre de Andrade" General Hospital, Habana Vieja, Havana City, Cuba

Abstract

The Kaposi's Sarcoma (KS) has acquired a relevant clinical importance in the past 20 years because it is a malignant tumor frequently associated with HIV infection. It is a multifocal vascular lesion of low-grade malignancy that typically appears on the skin of the lower extremities. The internal organs and lymph nodes are damaged less frequently. More rarely involve muscles, the Central Nervous System, peripheral nerves, heart, breast, salivary glands and the eyes.

---

* MD. Internal Medicine department "Freyre de Andrade" General Hospital. Internal Medicine Professor. 1-Morro 58 street between Genios and Refugio. Habana Vieja. Havana City. Cuba zip code: 10100. phone: 53-7-8639812 E-mail: roberto.albin@infomed.sld.cu.
** MD. Clinical Pathology department "Freyre de Andrade" General Hospital. Pathology Professor. phone: 53-7-2624752 E-mail: jccardenas@infomed.sld.cu.

Approximately 60% of the KS are presented with purple nodular lesions on the skin and/or of the oral mucosa. The other 40% has visceral injury with involvement of the gastrointestinal tract or invasion of the lungs. The disease can take in these cases with bleeding, perforations and obstruction. When there is a commitment to gastrointestinal tract, endoscopic study shows purple nodular lesions characteristic on the way from the mucosa. The differential diagnosis includes the hemangioma, bacillary angiomatosis, Blue Rubber Bleb Nevus Syndrome, the Osler-Weber-Rendu disease, Klippel-Trenaunay Syndrome and von Hippel-Lindau disease. That is why we need an accurate histopathological diagnosis in order to confirm the KS. The Immunohistochemistry staining for the virus HHV-8 have a 95-98% sensitivity and 100% specificity for the KS lesions. Other studies of Immunohistochemistry do not less important are the staining for CD31, CD34, CD40, Ki67, alpha Actin (SMA) and D2-40. The purpose of this chapter is to highlight the importance of maintaining a high clinical suspicion of the disease when the doctor faced with symptoms and signs that is studying the disease. On the other hand, the doctor must know the different diagnostic tools that are currently in clinical pathology in order to confirm this disease and thus engage in misdiagnosis, due the implications for the physical and mental health to which leads to the confirmation of the diagnosis of the KS. We intend to encourage the learning of all the clinical syndromes of presentation of the KS as well as the importance of the accurate diagnosis by immunohistochemical methods.

Introduction

Kaposi's Sarcoma(KS) is a multifocal vascular tumor of low-intermediate malignant grade that was first described by Moritz Kaposi, a Hungarian dermatologist, in 1872 as "idiopathic multiple pigmented sarcomas of the skin" and has been linked to human herpes virus 8 (HHV-8), a gamma-herpes virus [1]. There are four epidemiologic forms of KS and they have different trends and prognostic:

- Classic KS or Mediterranean,
- African or endemic KS
- Organ transplant-associated KS or iatrogenic, and
- AIDS-associated or epidemic KS.

The classic variant of KS primarily affects men (male: female ratio of 7:1) who are older with a mean age of 74 years and of Eastern European or Mediterranean descent. Lesions present as symmetric, harden, purple or reddish-brown macules, plaques, and nodules that appear primarily on the lower extremities. The involvement of internal organs and lymph nodes is rare, and their primary compromise is even more uncommon.

African or endemic KS is an aggressive form that is widespread among immunocompetent children and young adults in Equatorial Africa. It is often found in South Africa in young Bantu children [2, 3]. Nodules and plaques on edematous limbs are common in adults but rare in children. Visceral and lymphatic involvements are frequent too.

Organ transplant-associated KS or iatrogenic occurs in transplant recipients receiving immunosuppressive therapy and is very aggressive. The median time extend across transplant to KS diagnosis is about 2½ years.

AIDS-associated KS is the most aggressive form and is most prevalent in men who have sex with men, although recently, the implicate demographics have become more heterogeneous. HIV patients with CD4 counts between 200-500/cu mm have been affected most frequently by KS. Lesions present on the skin and visceral organs, especially the lungs and gastrointestinal tract. KS in an HIV patient is considered an AIDS-defining condition, according to the Centers for Disease Control and Prevention (CDC) Guidelines. KS is over 20,000-100,000 times more common in persons with AIDS than in the general population and over 300 times more common than in other immunosuppressed patients, such as renal transplant recipients [2, 3, 4, 5].

As HHV-8 has been detected in all four forms of Kaposi sarcoma (Kaposi's sarcoma-associated herpes virus: KSHV), these forms likely represent different manifestations of the same pathologic process. The disease begins as a reactive polyclonal angioproliferative response against this virus, in which polyclonal cells transform to oligoclonal cells that expand and undergo malignant changes. Genes encoded by this viral DNA have the potential to provoke cellular proliferation and prevent apoptosis. HHV-8 infection of endothelial cells or circulating mononuclear cells or haematopoietic progenitors leads to changes in their morphology, glucose metabolism, growth rate, lifespan and gene expression, resulting in the occurrence of KS. Most people infected with HHV-8 do not get Kaposi's sarcoma; the cancer appears most frequently when a person with HHV-8 also has a lowered immune system. HHV-8 has also been implicated in Cattleman's disease and non-Hodgkin's effusion lymphoma. HHV-8 and its relationship with KS was discovered by Chang et al. in 1994[6].

Clinical Symptoms

Classic KS or Mediterranean (CKS)

This occurs most often in older men (> 60 yr) of Italian, Jewish, Eastern European or Middle Eastern ancestry. However, ethnic features are not a rule and depend on the region or country. Kim M Hiatt et al. found a prevailingly of Caucasian/American (56%) in a study that included 438 non-HIV-related Kaposi Sarcoma patients while Mediterranean ethnic was 22% , South American Hispanic (18%), Black (10%), western European (4%), Middle East (4%). However, in North America, Classic Kaposi Sarcoma is rare with an incidence of 2.6–4.1 per million men and 0.6–0.9 per million women compared with incidences as high as 50/million men and 28/million women in rural areas of Italy and 16.9/million men and 6.3/million women in Israel [7].

Classic KS has an indolent course, and the disease is usually confined to a small number of lesions on the skin of the lower extremities. Over 70% of the Classic Kaposi Sarcoma patients have solitary lesions, 20% have multifocal disease, and <10% have disseminated disease. Patients with AIDS-related Kaposi Sarcoma have a higher percentage of multifocal (80%) and disseminated disease.

KS lesions are typically papular or nodular from several millimeters to centimeters in diameter (up to 15 cm) but median range of 1.5 cm. Nodules may be umblicated. Less commonly, KS lesions may be plaque-like or macula, especially on the thighs and soles of the feet, and sometimes they are ulcerated. Macules become papules, plaques, nodules, and tumors. Lesions may be pink, brown, red and purples or violaceous. Lesions are palpable, feeling firm to hard and may initially occur at sites of trauma, usually in the limbs. Oedema occurs along with these lesions principally on lower extremities. Other clinical features include infiltrative, telangiectatic, keloidal, ecchymotic, and lymphangioma-like or cavernous KS [1,3,7]

The few reported cases of classic KS with lymph node involvement have been presented in retrospective series and they don't mention clinical features. Hbid et al. reported 19 cases of CKS for a period of one year, none with lymph node compromise. Dal Maso et al. reported 874 cases of CKS obtained from 15 records of cancer during 1985-1998 and they found 27 cases (4.3%) located in subcutaneous tissue and other soft tissues. Dilnur et al. reported 17 cases of Classic KS during 1983-1998, and only one of them got lymph nodes compromise widespread, without dermal commitment. Stratigos et al. reported

66 patients with CKS during a period of 5 years (1990-1995), and 10 (15.5%) cases with lymph node compromise. They recognized that amount was high as regards to other series and did not mention if the lesions were primary or presented dermal involvement associate. García et al reviewed data of 79 patients with CSK during 1935-1985 and found 4 with lymph node involvement cases (3 inguinal and 1 popliteal). Kim M Hiatt et al. found 6 cases (1%) with lymph node compromise from 438 patients. S Mohanna et al. reported 3 patients with this condition: 1 of them began with growth of inguinal lymph node and later developed skin disease. The other 2 cases presented skin lesions along with palpable peripheral axilar and inguinal lymph nodes. This report did described clinical features. There are not data about the course or outcome in patients with lymph node compromise except in the report of S Mohanna et al. where two patients died early [4,8,9, 10,11,12].

As a rule, in CKS, the lymph node involvement is a rare condition (inguinal lymph nodes involvement is the most frequent presentation) and may be associated to poor survival.

Visceral involvement occurs in < 10%. This form is usually not fatal. Nevertheless, it had been reported patients with aggressive behavior of classical Kaposi's sarcoma. Gambassi et al. reported a case with CKS and severe gastrointestinal involvement that died into the first year from the diagnostic. Even in its classical form, KS may be a malignant, fulminant tumor. The extent and rate of spread of initial skin lesions should be considered to be early signs of aggressive dissemination. There are other variables to consider associated with worsening of the disease: histological pattern and human herpes virus type 8 positive in peripheral mononuclear cells [13]. Also, CKS may be associated to another tumors like angiosarcoma, Hodgkin lymphoma, non-Hodgkin lymphoma, myeloma multiple and chronic lymphocytic leukemia.

African or Endemic KS

In 1959 was described a second endemic variety in Equatorial Africa, affecting particularly children and young men. This form of Kaposi's sarcoma was very aggressive with visceral involvement and coursed almost fulminant. Nowadays, it represents almost half of all malignancies of Kenya and Nigeria.

This form occurs in Equatorial or sub-Sahara Africa independent of HIV infection. There are two types:

- *Prepubertal lymphadenopathic* form: It often affects children; primary tumors involve lymph nodes, with or without skin lesions. Lymphadenopathy may be local or generalized. The course is usually aggressive and fatal due to early involvement of internal organs.
- *Adult form*: This form courses with skin disease that resembles classic KS.

Endemic KS occurs more often in adults, but has been reported to be more aggressive in children [14].

Organ Transplant-Associated KS or Iatrogenic

Kaposi sarcoma is 150 to 200 times more likely to develop in people who have received an organ transplant than in the general population. This form develops between several months to several years after organ transplantation with immunosuppressive therapy. Lesions develop on the skin. Mucosal, lymph node, and visceral involvement occurs in about half of patients, even in the absence of skin lesions or preceding the development of these lesions. The course is more or less fulminant, depending on the degree of immunesuppression.

AIDS-Associated or Epidemic KS

It is the most common type of Kaposi sarcoma. This is the most common AIDS-associated malignancy and is more aggressive than Classic KS. Sometimes KS is the first sign of AIDS. AIDS-associated Kaposi sarcoma has no preferred locations but is widely spread, and involvement of the lymph nodes and intestine occurs relatively early. In most cases, visceral involvement carries a worse prognosis and accounts for approximately 40%-50% of overall cases. AIDS-associated KS tends to be multifocal (80%), often involving mucous membranes along the entire gastrointestinal tract and occurring in *atypical locations*.

Skin: Multiple cutaneous lesions are typically present, often involving the face and trunk. Skin lesions features have a similar appearance to classic KS ones.

Oral cavity Lesions on palate inside oral cavity are common, appearing in one third of cases and in the 15% as the first disease symptom. Oral KS could present initially as well delimited, painless, brownish, red to purple macule or papule. It could appear as a single or multiple lesions with dimensions varying in diameter from millimeters to centimeters, increasing slowly in size, forming nodules with or without ulceration. KS lesions could bleed and infiltrate bone and provoke tooth mobility [15]. Gingiva is affected too. In adults, AIDS-associated KS tends to be more aggressive, and oral cavity lesions along with visceral involvement are common.

Lymphatic system: In a series of Ugandan children with epidemic KS, lymph node involvement was observed in the majority of cases. Lymphadenopathic KS appeared to be a clinical presentation, which tended to occur in younger children and at higher CD4 T-cell counts [14].

Although lymphatic obstruction and lymphedema are frequent features of KS in HIV-infected adults, prominent lymph node involvement has been reported less often. Lymphedema is a common sign, particularly in the lower extremities and genitalia and may be incommensurate to the extent of skin disease and may be caused both to obliteration of lymphatics by KS and to the effects of cytokines like vascular endothelial growth factor (*VEGF*) involved in the pathogenesis of KS. The course is fatal too [14,16].

GI: Kaposi sarcoma is the most common gastrointestinal malignancy in AIDS. Approximately, 40% of patients have gastrointestinal (GI) tract involvement at initial diagnosis [3,16]. When gastrointestinal involvement is present, the endoscopic images are characteristics (nodular purple lesions or umbilicated nodule with central ulceration) but some cases resemble polypoid lesions. We reported a case with this endoscopic image [17]. Lesions may be extended to esophagus, stomach, duodenum and jejunum. Anemia could be present due to gastrointestinal bleeding. Bleeding could be imperceptible. GI lesions may cause abdominal pain, nausea and vomiting, malabsorption, or diarrhea. Perforation and obstruction of the bowel have been reported too.

Despite GI damaged, patients may be asymptomatic for a long time. Autopsy reveals 80% of GI involvement in the overall of AIDS-associated KS.

Liver involvement occurs only in epidemic KS and is usually associated with KS lesions in another site. Liver lesions are seen in 12 to 25% of fatal cases in this population. The KS tumors are multiple, varying in size from millimeters to 7-cm nodules, appearing red-brown, spongiform, hemorrhagic, portal in location, but sometimes infiltrating the adjacent parenchyma [18].

Pulmonary involvement generally occurs in severely immunosupressed patients who already have mucocutaneous or digestive involvement. Pulmonary involvement is also common and may present as shortness of breath, fever (as a common symptom), non-productive cough, hemoptysis, or chest pain or as an asymptomatic finding on chest x-ray examination. Pleural effusion may be present. Physical examination of the thorax is usually normal, but non-specific signs such as crackles, wheezing, and stridor may be present [19]. Computed tomography scan of the chest can show pulmonary nodules, interstitial or alveolar infiltrates; pleural effusion, and hilar or mediastinal lymphadenopathy. The most frequent CT finding is interstitial thickening, involving the peribronchovascular layers, often beginning in the peri-hilar regions and then progressing to the periphery. The peribronchovascular thickening may provoke irregular narrowing of the bronchial lumen by mucous lesions. Bronchoscopy may be show violaceous nodular or macular lesions in the patient's upper trachea and/or bronchi. Endobronchial lesions may narrow and partially obstruct the airways. Pulmonary disease occurs in 6%–32% of HIV patients who have skin manifestations of Kaposi sarcoma and is associated with a median survival of 1½ years and a 5-year overall survival rate of 50% [16,19,20]. We assisted a 16 years old patient with pulmonary infiltrate and severe right pleural effusion who died 2 months later. Sometimes, KS pulmonary diagnosis is very difficult because of its association to *Pneumocystis jirovecii (karinii)* pneumonia. Around 15% of patients with pulmonary KS may have no evidence of cutaneous KS. The subgroup of patients with pulmonary involvement gets the most unfavorable survival rate.

The *psychosocial* aspects concerning to KS are emotional distress, isolation, anger, loss of employment and guilt [21].

Epidemic KS has a highly variable clinical course, ranging from minimal disease presenting as an incidental finding to rapid growth resulting in a high morbidity and mortality.

Clinical Features in Unusual Presentations of KS

Medical publications have reported the appearance of KS in many unusual sites.

Gastrointestinal; rare involvement include primary KS of the appendix (One case of HIV-related Kaposi sarcoma of the appendix and acute appendicitis has been described in the literature) [22], isolated rectal KS, and KS with mesenteric localization [23].

Nervous System (CNS): Few cases of brain involvement with KS have been reported. All epidemiologic forms of KS may present CNS involvement. KS has been reported principally in the cerebrum, but has been found also in the cerebellum, pons, meninges and dura mater. CNS invasion is almost always seen within widespread KS disease. Symptoms of presentation may be seizures and hemiparesis. On Computer Tomography scan, KS appears as hyperdense lesions with edema and minimal mass effect. On MRI, brain KS lesions also appear as a homogeneous mass, of high signal intensity with T2 WI [23]. These clinical symptoms and radiologic findings were described in few cases.

Spinal cord involvement is a rare presentation of KS disease because only 2 cases have been reported with KS infiltrating the spinal cord. Symptoms were acute paraparesia, radicular pain, back pain, and tenderness over the thoracic and lumbar spine [23,24]. On MRI (Magnetic Resonance Image) spine, were found abnormal enhancement or high signal intensity with T2 weighted sequence in multiple thoracic and lumbar vertebrae (figure 1)

Peripheral nerve involvement by KS is rare: Only one case had been reported with KS infiltrating lumbar spinal cord, sacral plexus, sciatic and femoral nerves.

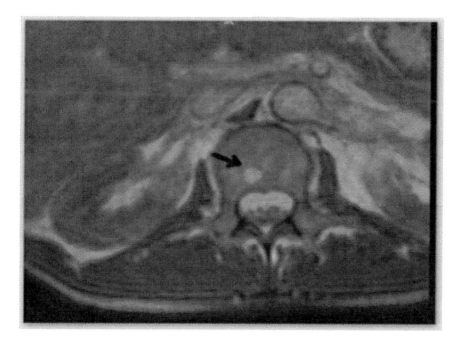

Figure 1. MRI Hyper intense Lesion WT2 in Patient with KS and Radicular Pain.

Larynx: Symptoms may include hoarseness, throat discomfort, dry cough, aphonia, dysphagia, stridor or complete airway obstruction. On examination, we may find laryngeal edema or a purple umblicated nodule. The lesion's surface can appear verrucous due to deposits of dry secretion. The diagnosis can be done by laryngoscopy or radiology studies. CT scan of the larynx may be useful. Biopsy is a key for diagnosis but dangerous because it has been implicated with fatal bleeding[23].

Thoracic duct: Pleural effusion with diagnosis of chylothorax is produced by development of in-situ KS in the thoracic duct[23].

Eyes: Ocular KS is rare (0.1-0.25%), although it may be the first manifestation of HIV infection. KS of the conjunctiva and ocular adnexa has been reported in association with Classic and AIDS-related KS. Conjunctiva lesions may be seen in any part of the palpebral or bulbar conjunctiva but are usually more common in the inferior fornix. Symptoms of presentation are: slight to mild pain in eyelids(most frequently in the inferior eyelid) as a result of hemorrhagic nodules in the inferior eyelid; a mass lesion or a conjunctiva haemorrhage; epiphora (overflow of tears) due to KS of the nasolacrimal duct; and, periorbital edema may occur with KS of the face or orbit [17,23]. Kaposi's sarcoma in the conjunctiva can be mistaken for a conjunctiva hemorrhage or pyogenic granuloma, papilloma, epidermoid carcinoma, and melanoma [25,26].

Musculoskeletal system: It is a rare site of KS occurrence. Seventy cases have been reported. Within the musculoskeletal system, KS lesions of bones are more frequently encountered than KS in skeletal muscle.

Four epidemiologic form have been involved with this rare manifestation of KS, and is most infrequently in organ transplant-associated KS. Medical literature reviewal made by Liron Pantanowitz and Bruce J Dezube published on 2008 found only one case with osseous involvement in a female patient with iatrogenic KS.

African and CKS lesions tend to involve the peripheral skeleton, whereas AIDS-related KS more commonly involves the axial skeleton (vertebrae, ribs, sternum, and pelvis) and maxillofacial bones. KS has been diagnosed in just about everything bones of the body (skull, maxilla, hard palate and mandible, vertebrae, ribs, sternum, pelvis, humerus, radius, ulna, femur, tibia, fibula, metacarpals, talus, calcaneus, and metatarsals). Joint involvement is unusual, but has been reported too [23,27,28,29,30]. KS involvement of bone without KS disease elsewhere is an exception. Involvement of bone marrow, without any osseous lesion, is far more common in AIDS-related KS.

Symptoms more frequently observed could be local bone pain with limited mobility, acute spinal cord compression, and intraoral tumor mass. Asymptomatic forms may be present but are not seen frequently. Pathological fractures do not seem to be a problem. Few cases, all AIDS patients, have had primary intraosseous KS .Most of the cases with KS bone involvement had been caused by infiltrating adjacent primary mucosal or skin lesions.

CT (Computer Tomography) scan and MRI (Magnetic Resonance Image) appear to be superior for the detection of KS bone lesions to osseous X-rays. Lesions are osteolytics.

CD4+ T-cell count of <100 cells/mm3 is often seen in patients with AIDS-related KS and bone involvement.

Prognosis is very bad when muscle or bone involvement is presented.

Kidneys and bladder: Urinary system is rarely involved by KS. There are 3 cases reported (one with kidney involvement and three with bladder involvement), all of them with organ transplant-associated KS. Symptoms were hematuria and obstruction with urinary retention by urethral meatal lesions [31,32]

Breast: KS can present as a small deep palpable mass or as a skin lesion. One case was reported with *peau d'orange* appearance of the breast due to KS axillary lymphatic involvement [23,33].

Over 15-18% of the four epidemiologic forms of Kaposi Sarcoma patients had *Cardiac* involvement in autopsy (KS lesions on epicardium) but any heart symptom had been reported up to date[34].

Endocrine glands: adrenal KS have been published, mostly in patients with AIDS, and it is a frequent site of KS involvement but sometimes is asymptomatic. Chronic adrenal failure may be present. None cases of acute adrenal failure has been reported.

Involvement of the thyroid gland by KS is rare. Symptoms may be an asymptomatic thyroid nodule and hypothyroidism.

Trauma and scars: A few cases have been reported. Some authors believe that post-traumatic KS lesions represent the Koebner phenomenon (the appearance of a skin lesion as a result of trauma). It has been reported growing KS on surgical scar a short time after surgery. A patient with primary KS as a result of radiation of the head and neck was reported [35]. It has been reported KS on a dermatome previously damaged by herpes zoster [36].

Salivary glands: Patients with KS of their salivary glands have been reported to present a 1 cm to 4 cm mass or swelling of the major salivary gland.

Subcutaneous tissue: It was reported by Liron Pantanowitz et al one case of primary KS involvement of the subcutaneous tissue without KS disease elsewhere. An HIV-positive patient presented slowly enlarging mass in the proximal left anterior thigh. He described stabbing pain, often experiencing sharp shooting pains down the left thigh. MRI showed a solid, vascular enhancing mass with spiculated margins located within the subcutaneous fat, superficial to muscle, in the left anterior thigh. Tumor was isointense to muscle on T1WI and heterogeneous, but mostly hyperintense on T2WI[37].

For doctors it is of great importance to know the unusual presentations of the KS. KS behaves as a systemic disease and may cause of almost all organs of the human body. The knowledge of the clinical features derived from the appearance of KS from uncommon body sites will allow the healthcare professional more efficient diagnostic certainty.

Immune Reconstitution Inflammatory Syndrome (IRIS) and Kaposi's Sarcoma

Although the IRIS does not form part of the original clinical picture of the KS, we consider appropriate to bring it up the description because it may be a complication that may arouse confusion during the treatment of the KS.

The use of highly active antiretroviral therapy (HAART) has resulted in a great reduction in opportunistic infections, AIDS-defining illnesses (like KS), and mortality in patients with HIV infection. Many studies have demonstrated that starting HAART in the setting of advanced HIV infection may be associated with the reactivation of indolent infections, particularly Mycobacterium tuberculosis, Mycobacterium avium complex, Cryptococcus neoformans, Pneumocystits karinii pneumonia, and viral hepatitis in a process known as immune reconstitution inflammatory syndrome (IRIS). IRIS may be defined as a progressive deterioration in clinical status as a result of recovery of the immune system, leading to worsening infections despite improvements in surrogate markers of HIV. IRIS is thought to be the direct result of a reconstituted immune system recognizing pathogens or antigens that were previously present, but clinically asymptomatic. IRIS is associated with a wide range of clinical manifestations generally associated with the specific infection that reactivates [38,39].

KS is caused by a gamma-herpes virus, so is named Kaposi's Sarcoma–associated Herpesvirus (KSHV). IRIS is well recognized as a complication of infection with another herpesvirus, cytomegalovirus (CMV). HAART decreases KSHV viral load and the incidence of KS, increases the time to treatment failure in KS and, leads to heal isolated lesions. Thereby, a number of characteristics of AIDS-associated KS suggest that it is a probable disease for IRIS. M. Bower et al [40] demonstrated that KS can exacerbate during HAART-associated increases in the CD4 count and KS is an IRIS-associated disease. IRIS-KS was linked with a significantly higher CD4 count at the time of KS and diagnosis was associated with the specific infection that reactivates. M. Bower et al described a series of 10 patients with IRIS-related progression of KS from a cohort of 150 antiretroviral-naive patients with KS who started HAART. All ten patients developed new KS lesions and progression of established lesions during the first 2 months following the start of HAART. Authors observed a temporal relationship between rapid clinical deterioration of KS and the starting of HAART[40]. The small number of patients limited the results of this study but we believe that it should be taken into account when occurs a similar episode during the treatment of a patient affected with AIDS associated- KS.

Rule out

Lesions can be mistaken clinically for purpura, ecchymotic lesions, hematomas, angiomas, dermatofibromas, and red nevi.

Bacillary angiomatosis: It is an infectious disease and is presented by skin lesions usually tender, glistening, eroded papules and nodules; may exude serous or purulent discharge, closely resemble pyogenic granulomas, range from mm-cm in diameter; may appear as tender subcutaneous nodules or ulcerations, angiomatous papules. On physical examination we may find tender lymphadenopathy and subcutaneous and lytic bone lesions. Causes: Rochalimaea henselae, also called Bartonella henselae; Bartonella quintana. It is a slow-growing, gram-negative bacillus, which can be identified by Warthin-Starry silver .Risk factors: cat scratch or bite may be risk factor for bacillary angiomatosis/cat and flea exposure associated with B. henselae infection; while B. quintana infection associated with low income, homelessness and exposure to lice [41].

The differential diagnosis includes too:

Blue Rubber Bleb Nevus Syndrome: This syndrome is a disorder characterized by cavernous hemangiomas of the skin, soft-tissue, bones, and viscera. Also, the Blue Rubber Bleb Nevus Syndrome is associated with a variety of other disorders, including *Maffucci's syndrome* (skin and soft tissue hemangiomas and enchondromatosis), chronic lymphocytic leukemia and hypernephroma, disseminated intravascular coagulopathy, and *diffuse angiokeratoma* [42,43,44,45]

The following diseases have characteristic lesions and patterns of involvement muco-cutaneous, including: *Osler-Weber-Rendu disease* (multiple skin and mucosal membrane telangiectasias); *Klippel-Trenaunay syndrome* (vascular nevus of the lower limb, varicosities, osteohypertrophy and gastrointestinal angiomas); von *Hippel-Lindau disease* (retinal angiomas, cerebellar hemangioblastoma) and *ataxia-telangiectasia* (cerebellar ataxia, oculocutaneous telangiectasias, and immunodeficiency)

Diagnosis

A thorough physical examination of the patient must be performed with special attention in sites typically involved by KS, such as the lower extremities, face, oral mucosa, genitalia, lymphatic system, GI tract, and lungs.

In addition to a physical examination, the following tests may be used to diagnose Kaposi sarcoma:

- *Biopsy with inmunohistochemistry staining* for HHV-8, CD31, CD34, CD40, Ki67, alpha Actin and D2-40. It is especially important to obtain a biopsy of lesions. Other tests can suggest that KS is present, but only a biopsy can make a definite diagnosis.
- *HIV test/ Western Blot*
- *HIV-1 viral load:* It is essential for staging and for treatment the disease.
- $CD4^+$ *T-lymphocyte count:* It is essential for staging and for treatment the disease too.
- To determine if Kaposi Sarcoma has spread to internal organs, we may perform the following examinations:
- *Stools occult blood testing*: screening of GI tract lesions may be done by this lab exam.
- *X-ray:* A chest x-ray can help to determine if the cancer has spread to the lungs. Chest x-ray is an excellent means of screening for pulmonary lesions.
- *Computed tomography (CT or CAT) scan.* CT scans of the chest and abdomen can help find KS that has spread to the lungs, lymph nodes, or liver.
- *Endoscopy:* Endoscopy can be done in patients with occult blood or GI symptoms.
- *Bronchoscopy:* Bronchoscopy must be performed for cases with abnormal findings on a chest radiograph or CT and so patient with

unhealed respiratory symptoms when no other cause is found. The appearance of characteristic tracheobronchial KS lesions is considered enough to make a correct diagnosis of pulmonary KS.
- *Photography:* Because many skin lesions can appear in many body sites, doctors may get pictures from parts of the skin (called mapping) to find out if new lesions have developed over time.

Kaposi's Sarcoma Morphology

Regardless of the clinical form of KS, microscopic morphology of sarcoma of Sarcoma (KS) is going to be similar: a hemorrhagic sarcoma of intermediate degree of malignancy.

However, the distribution of the lesions varies according to the clinical presentation; Thus, they will may be located in the skin of the lower extremities as plaques or nodular, with insidious behavior, described classically by Kaposi. The lymphadenopathic form, also called African or endemic KS in which injuries are settled in lymph nodes (localized or generalized) along with visceral involvement. This form respects the skin, but is very aggressive or fulminant (prepubertal lymphadenopathic form).

With the advent of organ transplants in the second half of the last century and as a complication of immunosuppressive treatment, it was described a third form in recipients of organs, which has as characteristic, the combination of morphological alterations both in the skin and internal organs. This clinical form has the particularity of achieve a partial remit when immunosuppressive treatment is withdrawn, although in the end these transplant receptor patients will die by the spread of the tumor

From 1981, with the onset of AIDS was described the fourth clinical form, where it joins the distribution of these hemorrhagic sarcoma lesions described previously in the other three forms: lesions on skin of lower extremities and anywhere, including the lining of the eye and the mouth. This form curses with lymph nodes and viscera involvement, and a distribution of hemorrhagic nodules in the gastrointestinal tract [47].

Macroscopic and Microscopic Morphology

The hemorrhagic Kaposi's sarcoma usually evolves by three periods: the macula, the plaque and the nodule, which can be distinguished in the classic type.

This disease begins as a macula, which may be small and solitary or multiple. They may converge and become more extensive, located in the skin of the feet or the distal lower limb. They are pink at the beginning of its appearance, but eventually become reddish-purple. At this time, taking a sample for biopsy to microscopic examination we can find some elements that make us suspect its presence but indistinguishable from the components of the reparative granulation tissue, that is, a mixture of inflammatory cells (lymphocytes, macrophages with or without hemosiderin and plasma cells) with small dilated blood vessels, somewhat irregular and slightly prominent endothelial cells.

Evolutionarily these macules rise and become red-purplish plaques larger in size. When these plaques are observed with the optical microscope we can see, in the dermis, ducts and vascular splits of larger size than the macules, with jagged peaks and upholstered with thick spindle cells, but with the participation of a low-grade sarcomatous stroma, with few mitotic figures, among which appear scattered extravasated red blood cells (hemorrhage), hemosiderin from the destruction of these red blood cells and that is phagocytized by macrophages, lymphocytes and plasma cells. It may be find a few hyaline balloons of uncertain origin.

As disease advance, plaques become neoplastic purple nodules and they may be umblicated (Figure 2). The cellular component of them are the same but more pronounced than before. It is not only confined to the dermis, but extends to the subcutaneous tissue.

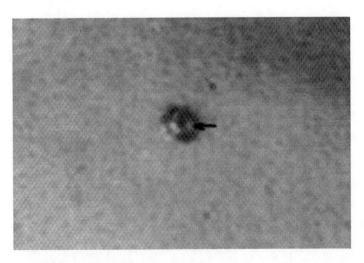

Figure 2. Umblicated Purple Nodule in KS Patient.

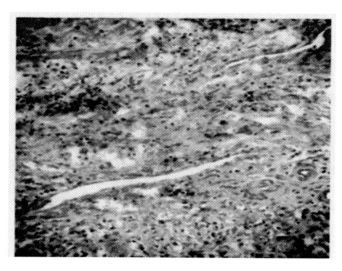

Figure 3. Histopathologic findings in KS associated to AIDS. Vascular proliferation, hemorrhage, spindle cells.

The proliferation of small vessels is accompanied by the lymph node and visceral involvement result in more aggressive clinical forms. Vessels are scattered and intermixed with splits and rows or clusters of spindle cells with increasing numbers of mitosis, as well as with intense hemorrhage, increased amount of hemosiderin, intracytoplasmic hyaline globules and blood cells, lymphocytes and macrophages (Nodular Stage) (Figure 3)

The origin of the proliferating spindle cells in Kaposi sarcoma is uncertain, though these cells are currently believed to be derived from lymphatic endothelium.

Immunohistochemistry shows expression of CD34, CD31, and D2-40 [3,17,48]. Another lymphatic endothelial cell marker (hyaluronan receptor LYVE-1), expressed by endothelial cells of normal lymphatic vessels but not blood vessels, is positive in angiosarcomas and Kaposi sarcomas. A monoclonal antibody (FHI-1) against the carboxyl terminal end of the FLI-1 protein can be reliably applied in the differential diagnosis of tumors of endothelial differentiation. All rhabdomyosarcomas, desmoplastic small round cell tumors, high-grade pleomorphic sarcomas, and colonic adenocarcinomas are negative for FLI-1. Therefore, FLI-1 can help in the differential diagnosis of nonvascular tumors such as gastrointestinal stromal tumors. Infection with HHV-8 is necessary for the development of Kaposi sarcoma in HIV patients, and, at present, it is considered the definitive cause of Kaposi sarcoma. Over 95-98% of Kaposi sarcoma lesions, regardless of their clinical form, have been found to be infected with HHV-8. The long-lasting expression of HHV-8 latency genes is important for Kaposi sarcoma spindle-cell progression [3,49,50]

In the following table we show the panel of immunohistochemical studies (IHC) most commonly used on Sarcoma, spindle cell tumors and other soft tissue injuries and results in KS, especially SMA (Figure 4), CD-34 (Figure 5) and Ki 67 also in mitosis (Figure 6)

Immunohistochemical studies for Kaposi's Sarcoma

Negative	Positive
AE1/AE3	SMA/ Ki 67
CAM 5.2	CD-34
EMA	CD-31
S-100	F VIII
HHF-35	FLI-1
DESMIN	HHV8
CD-117	D2-40

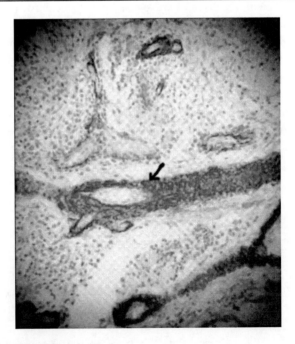

Figure 4. Alpha actin in blood vessels.

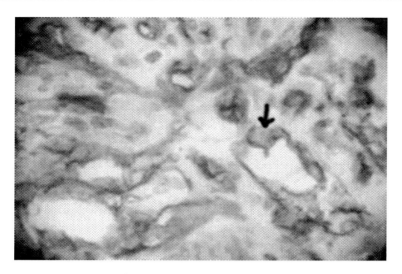

Figure 5. CD34 positive in KS associated to AIDS.

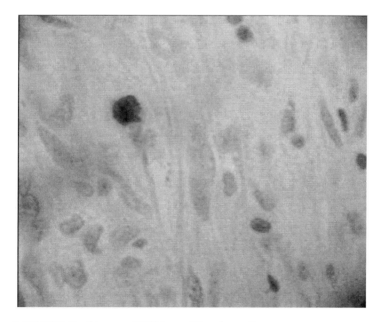

Figure 6. KS IHQ. Positive test Ki67 in proliferative cells.

AIDS-Related KS Staging System

The staging system for AIDS-related KS developed by the AIDS Clinical Trials Group (ACTG) of the NIH is the most used. It is as follow [16,51]:

	Good risk (all of the following)	Poor risk (any of the following)
Tumor(T)	Confined to skin and/or lymph nodes and/or minimal oral disease (no nodular KS confined to palate)	Tumor-associated edema or ulceration. Extensive oral KS. KS of GI tract KS in other non-lymph nodal viscera
Immune system(I)	CD4+ cell count >= 200 /µl	CD4+ cell count <200 /µl
Systemic illness(S)	No history of opportunistic infection or thrush "B" symptoms absent. Karnofsky performance status>=70	History of opportunistic infection and/or thrush "B" symptoms present. Karnofsky performance status<70 Other HIV-related illness(e.g. neurologic disease, lymphoma)

"B" symptoms are: unexplained fever, night sweats, weight loss >10%, diarrhea more than 2 weeks.

Prognosis

There are 4 factors predict mortality in AIDS-associated Kaposi sarcoma [52]:
Prognostic score (0-15); starts with 10 points;

- -3 points if Kaposi sarcoma was AIDS-defining illness
- +3 points if simultaneous AIDS-associated illness
- +2 points if age 50 years or older
- -1 point for every complete 100 cells/mm3 in CD4 count

Predicted survival:

- if 0 points - 99.3% at 1 year and 98.4% at 5 years
- if 5 points - 96.7% at 1 year and 91.8% at 5 years
- if 10 points - 83.4% at 1 year and 63.1% at 5 years
- if 15 points - 37.8% at 1 year and 8.4% at 5 years

Treatment

Aim of this chapter is not to deepen in the treatment of the KS, but we believe this review incomplete if we do not make a brief presentation on the current trends of the treatment.

The KS treatment depends on the clinical form and stage of disease at the time of diagnosis. The skin disease has multiple options treatment including surgical excision of lesions localized or unique. Cryosurgery, laser therapy and radiation therapy are therapeutic options.

Chemotherapeutics are very useful in the visceral commitment and systemic disease. It is the best treatment in these cases. Vinblastine alone or together with vincristine may be used by intravenous route. This combination can be effective in patients with AIDS-associated KS. The combination of vinblastine and bleomycin may be effective, especially in patients with CKS. Bleomycin can also be used alone to treat the disease. Other options include the following chemotherapy: liposomal doxorrubicin IV, blenoxane, etoposide, dacarbazine, actinomycin D and paclitaxel[53].

- intralesional vincristine reported to be associated with complete response in most treated lesions.
- alitretinoin 0.1% gel FDA approved for topical treatment of cutaneous AIDS-related Kaposi sarcoma; applied twice daily with gradual increase to 4 times daily if necessary.
- The immunotherapy is also an important aspect of the treatment of the KS. It has been shown the regression of the AIDS - associated KS with the use of highly active antiretroviral therapy or HAART.
- Systemic therapy with interferon alpha is used in the KS (slow or reverse KS in patients with CD4>400).

The reduction of immunosuppression achieves a reduction of 50% of the disease, especially in the skin forms. The introduction of highly active antiretroviral therapy (HAART) has radically changed the clinical course of human immunodeficiency virus (HIV) infection to reduce its impact by 10% over 1994.

- Antiretrovirals may help decrease the proportion of new lesions, promote regression of existing lesions, and improve survival with or without chemotherapy.
  Treatment of immune reconstitution inflammatory syndrome (IRIS) [54]
- Optimize or initiate treatment of underlying opportunistic infection.
- No specific treatment for IRIS needed if mild or limited to cutaneous disease.
- Nonsteroid anti-inflammatory drugs (NSAIDs) may be adequate for IRIS of moderate severity.
- Severe IRIS may require anti-inflammatory or immunomodulatory medications.
- Prednisone may reduce morbidity in patients with TB-IRIS.
- other treatments with efficacy in case reports include pentoxifylline, montelukast, thalidomide, hydroxychloroquine and infliximab ,
- interruption of antiretroviral therapy only considered for life-threatening IRIS

Conclusion

In conclusion, KS is a vascular tumor of lymphatic vessels of low-intermediate malignant grade. KS may have a viral origin because the gamma herpesvirus-8(HHV-8) has been identified at 95-98% of all the KS tumor lesions. It has four clinical forms. The most aggressive forms are lymphadenopathic of African children, the iatrogenic, and especially, AIDS-associated KS. It is a multifocal disease although some authors consider that demonstrations of lesions in unusual sites are rather expression of metastasis, i.e., the presence of lesions on the eyes and the brain. The course is very variable from an ill person to another, is heavily dependent on the degree of immunosuppression and spread of the disease. The more often clinical symptoms are skin lesions at any structure of the body, gastrointestinal symptoms, increase in lymph nodes and pulmonary symptoms. However, the clinical picture may be very broad because cases with condition of almost all organ systems have been reported. It is of great importance the knowledge of the symptoms and signs of the KS for all medical specialties because with the advent of the AIDS, KS turned from being a very rare disease to be the most common malignant tumor in patients with AIDS, and, doctors of all specialties are facing every day patients potentially carriers or patients with HIV. We must remember where the AIDS epidemic is global. In my clinical experience, many patients come with symptoms caused by KS without knowing that they are suffering from AIDS and, it is when the disease becomes more difficult to diagnose because the AIDS-associated KS occurs occasionally with involvement of internal organs and in turn with very few if any involvement of the skin. There are many diagnostic procedures to study KS, but only the biopsy confirms. The advent of immunohistochemistry has permitted a more accurate identification of the tumor through expression of CD34, CD31, Alpha Act, D2-40 and FLI-1but above all to be positive to HHV-8. New advances in its therapeutic have improved the prognosis and the incidence of this disease, but we must be alert to recognize secondary symptoms to the appearance of the IRIS in patient undergoing HAART for presenting an AIDS-associated KS.

References

[1] Goldenberg G, MD. A 35-Year-Old Man With Kaposi's Sarcoma. April 4,2009 [cited 2011 June 01]. Available from: http://www.medscape.com/viewarticle/590169.

[2] Korman A, MD; Favila K, DO; Wang L, MD; McCabe E, MD;. Carr-Locke D L, MD. Kaposi's Sarcoma of the Upper Gastrointestinal Tract Causing Severe Anemia. August 24,2010 [cited 2011 June 01]. Available from: http://www.medscape.com/ viewarticle/727175.

[3] Arora M, MD, Goldberg E M, MD. Kaposi Sarcoma Involving the Gastrointestinal Tract. *Gastroenterology and Hepatology* Volume 6, Issue 7 July 2010.

[4] Salim Mohanna B, Juvenal Sánchez L, Juan Carlos Ferrufino L, Francisco Bravo P, Eduardo Gotuzzo H. Sarcoma de Kaposi clásico ganglionar. Comunicación de tres casos. *Rev. Méd. Chile* 2007; 135: 1166-1170.

[5] Solivetti FM, Elia F, Latini A, Cota C, Cordiali-Fei P, Di Carlo A. AIDS-Kaposi Sarcoma and Classic Kaposi Sarcoma: are different ultrasound patterns related to different variants?. *Journal of Experimental and Clinical Cancer Research* 2011, 30:40.

[6] Chang Y, Cesarman E, Pessin MS, Lee F, Culpepper J, Knowles DM, et al. Identification of herpervirus-like DNA sequences in AIDS-associated Kaposis sarcoma. *Science* 1994;266:1865-9.

[7] Hiatt KM, Nelson AM, Lichy JH, Fanburg-Smith JC. Classic Kaposi Sarcoma in the United States over the last two decades: A clinicopathologic and molecular study of 438 non-HIV-related Kaposi Sarcoma patients with comparison to HIV-related Kaposi Sarcoma. *Modern Pathology* (2008) 21, 572–582.

[8] Hbid O, Belloul L, Fajali N, Ismaili N, Duprez R, Tanguy M et al. Kaposi's sarcoma in Morocco: a pathological study with immunostaining for human herpesvirus-8 *LNA-Pathology* 2005; 37: 288-95.

[9] Dal Maso L, Polesel J, Ascoli V, Zambon P, Budroni M, Ferretti S et al. Classic Kaposi's sarcoma in Italy, 1985-1998. *Br. J. Cancer* 2005; 92: 188-93.

[10] Dilnur P, Katano H, Wang ZH, Osakabe Y, Kudo M, Sata T et al. Classic type of Kaposi's sarcoma and human herpesvirus 8 infection in Xinjiang, China. *Pathol. Int.* 2001; 51: 845-52.

[11] Stratigos JD, Potouridou I, Katoulis AC. Classic Kaposi's sarcoma in Greece: a clinico-epidemiological profile. *Int. J. Dermatol.* 1997; 36: 735-40.

[12] Weissmann A, Linn S, Weltfriend S, Friedmanbirnbaum R. Epidemiological study of classic Kaposi's sarcoma: a retrospective review of 125 cases from Northern Israel. *J. Eur. Acad. Dermatol. Venereol.* 2000; 14: 91-5.

[13] Gambassi G, Semeraro R, Suma V, Sebastio A, Incalzi RA. Aggressive behavior of classical Kaposi's sarcoma and coexistence with angiosarcoma. *J. Gerontol. A Biol. Sci. Med. Sci.* 2005 Apr;60(4):520-3 [pubmed].

[14] Gantt S, MD PhD1,2, Kakuru A, MBChB3,4, Wald A, MD MPH2, Walusansa V, MBChB MMed. Corey L, MD, Casper C, MD MPH and Orem J, MBChB MMed. Clinical Presentation and Outcome of Epidemic Kaposi Sarcoma in Ugandan Children. *Pediatr. Blood Cancer.* 2010 May ; 54(5): 670–674. doi:10.1002/pbc.22369.

[15] Mohanna S, Bravo F, Ferrufino J C, Sanchez J, Gotuzzo E. Classic Kaposis sarcoma presenting in the oral cavity of two HIV-negative Quechua patients. *Med. oral patol. oral cir. (Internet)* vol.12 no.5 Madrid Sept. 2007.

[16] Dezube BJ, MD; Pantanowitz L, MD; Aboulafia DM, MD. Management of AIDS-Related Kaposi Sarcoma: *Advances in Target Discovery and Treatment.* June 2, 2004 [cited 2011 June 01]. Available from: http://www.medscape.com/viewarticle/479015.

[17] Cano, R. G. A. and Cardenas, J. C. P. (2011), Conjunctival metastasis from Kaposi's sarcoma: A case report. *Diagnostic Cytopathology*, 39: 128–131. doi: 10.1002/dc.21381.

[18] Bioulac-Sage P; Laumonier H; Laurent C; Blanc JF; Balabaud C.Benign and Malignant Vascular Tumors of the Liver in Adults. Dec 19,2008 *.Liver Dis.* 2008;28(3):302-314. © 2008 Thieme Medical Publishers [cited 2011 June 01]. Available from: http://www.medscape.com /viewarticle/584478Semin.

[19] Taisa Davaus Gasparetto, Edson Marchiori, Sílvia Lourenço, Gláucia Zanetti, Alberto Domingues Vianna1, Alair ASMD Santos ,Luiz Felipe Nobre. Pulmonary involvement in Kaposi sarcoma: correlation between imaging and pathology. *Orphanet Journal of Rare Diseases* 2009, 4:18 doi:10.1186/1750-1172-4-18. Available from: http://www.ojrd.com/ content/4/1/18.

[20] Kim C, Shu D. Kaposi sarcoma of the lung. *CMAJ.* 2008 July 1; 179(1): 107. doi: 10.1503/cmaj.071657. [cited 2011 June 03]. Available from: http://www.ncbi.nlm.nih.gov/pmc/articles/ 4481/?tool=pmcentrez.

[21] Holland JC, Tross S. Psychosocial considerations in the therapy of epidemic Kaposi's sarcoma. *Semin. Oncol.* 1987;14(2 suppl 3):48-53.

[22] Egwuonwu S, MD; Gatto-Weis C, MD; Miranda R, MD; De Las Casas L, MD. Gastrointestinal Kaposi Sarcoma with Appendiceal Involvement. May 05,2011[cited 2011 June 03] *South Med. J.* 2011;104(4):278-281. © 2011 Lippincott Williams and Wilkins. Available from: http://www.medscape.com/viewarticle/740974.

[23] Pantanowitz L and Dezube BJ, Kaposi sarcoma in unusual locations. BMC Cancer 2008, 8:190 doi:10.1186/1471-2407-8-190

[24] van Twillert G, van Eeden S, Nellen FJB, Cornelissen M, Wszolek Z, Westermann AM: Spinal cord compression due to Kaposi sarcoma. *Ann. Oncol.* 2004, 15:1143-4.

[25] Jyotirmay Biswas, MS and S Sudharshan, DO. Anterior segment manifestations of human immunodeficiency virus/acquired immune

deficiency syndrome. *Indian J. Ophthalmol.* 2008 Sep–Oct; 56(5): 363–375[PubMed].
[26] Mc Lean IW, Burnier MN et al. Tumors of the eye and ocular adnexa. *Atlas of tumor pathology.* Maryland: Advisor Board, 1994: 1 – 94[MEDLINE].
[27] Lausten LL, Ferguson BL, Barker BF, Cobb CM: Oral Kaposi sarcoma associated with severe alveolar bone loss: case report and review of the literature. *J. Periodontol.* 2003, 74:1668-75.
[28] Krishna G, Chitkara RK: Osseous Kaposi sarcoma. *JAMA* 2003, 289:1106.
[29] Thanos L, Mylona S, Kalioras V, Pomoni M, Batakis N: Osseous Kaposi sarcoma in an HIV-positive patient. *Skeletal. Radiol.* 2004, 33:241-3.
[30] Caponetti G, Dezube BJ, Restrepo CS, Pantanowitz L: Kaposi sarcoma of the musculoskeletal system. A review of 66 patients. *Cancer* 2007, March 15;109(6):1040-52.
[31] Biermann CW, Gasser TC, Rutishauser G: Kaposi sarcoma of theurinary bladder after kidney transplantation (article in German). *Helv. Chir. Acta* 1992, 59:503-5.
[32] Rha SE, Byun JY, Kim HH, Baek JH, Hwangm TK, Kangm SJ: Kaposi sarcoma involving a transplanted kidney, ureter and urinarybladder: ultrasound and CT findings. *Br. J. Radiol.* 2000, 73:1221-3.
[33] Ng CS, Taylor CB, O'Donnell PJ, Pozniak AL, Michell MJ: Case report: mammographic and ultrasound appearances of Kaposi sarcoma of the breast. *Clin. Radiol.* 1996, 51:735-6.
[34] Silver MA, Macher AM, Reichert CM, Levens DL, Parrillo JE, Longo DL, Roberts WC: Cardiac involvement by Kaposi sarcoma in acquired immune deficiency syndrome (AIDS). *Am. J. Cardiol.* 1984, 53:983-5.
[35] De Pasquale R, Nasca MR, Micali G: Postirradiation primary Kaposi sarcoma of the head and neck. *J. Am. Acad. Dermatol.* 1999, 40:312-4.
[36] Niedt GW, Prioleau PG: Kaposi sarcoma occurring in a dermatome previously involved by herpes zoster. *J. Am. Acad. Dermatol.* 1988, 18:448-51
[37] Pantanowitz L, Mullen J and Dezube BJ. Primary Kaposi sarcoma of the subcutaneous tissue. *World Journal of Surgical Oncology* 2008, 6:94 doi:10.1186/1477-7819-6-94.
[38] Autran B, Carcelain G, Debre P: Immune reconstitution after highly active anti-retroviral treatment of HIV infection. *Adv. Exp. Med. Biol.* 495:205-212, 2001[Medline].

[39] Shelburne SA 3rd, Hamill RJ, Rodriguez-Barradas MC, et al: Immune reconstitution inflammatory syndrome: Emergence of a unique syndrome during highly active antiretroviral therapy. *Medicine* (Baltimore) 81:213-227, 2002[Medline].
[40] Bower M, Nelson M, Young AM, Thirlwell C, Newsom-Davis T, Mandalia S, Dhillon T, Holmes P, Gazzard BG, Stebbing J. Immune Reconstitution Inflammatory Syndrome Associated With Kaposi's Sarcoma. *Journal of Clinical Oncology*, Vol 23, No 22 (August 1), 2005: pp. 5224-5228.
[41] Dynamed[internet site] Bacillary angiomatosis. June 06,2011[cited 2011 jun 06]. Available from: http://dynaweb.ebscohost.com/Detail?id= AN+116391andsid=8c818277-9913-48fe-a128-91ef580305cc@ sessionmgr111.
[42] Aihara M, Konuma Y, Okawa K, et al: Blue Rubber Bleb Nevus Syndrome with disseminated intravascular coagulation and thrombocytopenia: successful treatment with high-dose intravenous gamma globulin. *Tohoku J. Exp. Med.* 1991; 163:111-117[MEDLINE].
[43] Shimada S, Namikawa K, Maeda K, et al: Endoscopic polypectomy under laparotomy throughout the alimentary tract for a patient with Blue Rubber Bleb Nevus Syndrome. *Gastrointest. Endosc.* 1997; 45:423-427[MEDLINE].
[44] Kunishige M, Azuma H, Masuda K, et al: Interferon alpha-2a therapy for disseminated intravascular coagulation in a patient with Blue Rubber Bleb Nevus Syndrome: a case report. *Angiology* 1997; 48:273-277[MEDLINE].
[45] White CW, Sondheimer HM, Crouch EC, et al: Treatment of pulmonary hemangiomatosis with recombinant interferon alfa-2a. *N. Engl. J. Med.* 1989; 320:1197-1200[MEDLINE].
[46] Klippel M, Trenaunay P: Du noevus variqueux osteohypertrophique. *Arch. Gen. Med.* 1900; 185:641-672[MEDLINE].
[47] Kalpidis CD, Lysitsa SN, Lombardi T, Kolokotronis AE, Antoniades DZ, Samson J. Gingival Involvement in a Case Series of Patients with Acquired immunodeficiency syndrome-related Kaposi sarcoma. *J. Periodontol.* 2006 Mar; 77 (3) :523-33.
[48] Kahn HJ, Bailey D, Marks A. Monoclonal antibody D2-40, a new marker of lymphatic endothelium, reacts with Kaposi's sarcoma and a subset of angiosarcomas. *Mod. Pathol.* 2002;15:434-440.

[49] Xu H, Edwards JR, Espinosa O, Banerji S, Jackson DG, Athanasou NA. Expression of a lymphatic endothelial cell marker in benign and malignant vascular tumors. *Hum. Pathol.* 2004;35:857-861.

[50] Rossi S, Orvieto E, Furlanetto A, Laurino L, Ninfo V, Dei Tos AP. Utility of the immunohistochemical detection of FLI-1 expression in round cell and vascular neoplasm using a monoclonal antibody. *Mod. Pathol.* 2004;17:547-552.

[51] Krown SE, Metroka C, Wernz JC. Kaposi's sarcoma in the acquired immune deficiency syndrome: a proposal for uniform evaluation, response, and staging criteria. AIDS Clinical Trials Group Oncology Committee. *J. Clin. Oncol.* 1989;7:1201-1207.

[52] Stebbing J, Sanitt A, Nelson M, Powles T, Gazzard B, Bower M. A prognostic index for AIDS-associated Kaposi's sarcoma in the era of highly active antiretroviral therapy. *Lancet.* 2006 May 6;367(9521):1495-502.

[53] Aldenhoven M, Barlo NP, Sanders CJ. Therapeutic strategies for epidemic Kaposi's sarcoma. *Int. J. STD AIDS.* 2006;17:571-578. [MEDLINE].

[54] Dynamed[DataBase on Internet] Kaposi sarcoma;2011[cited 2011 March 06]; Available from: http://dynaweb.ebscohost.com/Detail?id= AN+115224andsid=5480217d-a67d-4692-ae57-b2981907912a@ sessionmgr11.

In: Sarcoma
Editor: Eric J. Butler

ISBN: 978-1-62100-362-5
© 2012 Nova Science Publishers, Inc.

Chapter III

M5076 Ovarian Sarcoma in Mice: Novel Chemotherapy by Drug Delivery System

Yasuyuki Sadzuka[*]

School of Pharmacy, Iwate Medical University,
2-1-1 Yahaba-Cho, Shiwa-Gun, Iwate, Japan

Abstract

M5076 ovarian sarcoma is transplantable murine reticulum sarcoma originating in ovary of C57BL/6 mice and highly invasive and metastatic. When M5076 ovarian sarcoma is s.c. transplanted onto the backs of mice, solid tumor arises, spontaneously metastasizes to the liver and lung, and then kills the mice within about 25-30 days. This sarcoma exhibited lower sensitivity to antitumor agent as doxorubicin (DOX). Namely, M5076 ovarian sarcoma which has high metastasis and resistance, induced unfavorable prognosis on host body. In current chemotherapy, it is important for treatment on the sarcoma of these profiles.

On biochemical modulation, the pharmacodynamics of antitumor agent is modulated by combination with another drug in order to enhance the antitumor activity or to reduce the adverse reaction, the

---

[*] Professor, School of Pharmacy, Iwate Medical University, 2-1-1 Yahaba-Cho, Shiwa-Gun, Iwate, 028-3694, Japan. E-mail : ysadzuka@iwate-med.ac.jp.

chemotherapic index is thereby enhanced. From these points, this concept is considered as drug delivery system. Theanine is specific amino acid and umami component in green tea. Theanine does not have antitumor activity whereas enhance some antitumor agents induced efficacy. Namely, the combination of theanine with non-effective dose of doxorubicin (DOX) suppressed M5076 ovarian sarcoma growing in vivo. In vitro, theanine inhibited DOX efflux from M5076 ovarian sarcoma cell and in vivo, combined theanine increased DOX concentration in the tumor without no change of DOX concentration in normal tissues in sarcoma bearing mice. From the evaluation in detail, the mechanism for the theanine induced effects speculated as follows. Some of the DOX taken up by M5076 ovarian sarcoma cells binds to glutathione (GSH) and thereby generates the GS-DOX conjugate. The conjugate is released extracellularly by the GS-X pump on M5076 ovarian sarcoma cells. Theanine suppressed the uptake of glutamate through inhibitions of GLAST and GLT-1 as glutamate transporters and thereafter reduced the biosynthesis of GSH in sarcoma cells. Then, generation of the conjugate of intracellular DOX and GSH is affected and the release of the GS-DOX conjugate by sarcoma cells via the MRP5/GS-X pump decrease.

On M5076 ovarian sarcoma cells, anserine and taurine as dipeptide, glutamate transporter inhibitors and methylxanthine derivatives enhanced antitumor activity of DOX, too. In conclusion, it is expected that the combination of food components and other agent with antitumor agent advances novel therapy on some sarcomas.

1. Introduction

In cancer chemotherapy, many antitumor agents have improved condition or symptom of cancer patients, whereas appearance of antitumor agent induced adverse reactions have damaged quality of life (QOL) of cancer patients. Namely, the applications of antitumor agents are double-edged sword in cancer chemotherapy. Furthermore, some sarcomas are intractable disease by a low sensitivity on the antitumor agents. M5076 ovarian sarcoma is transplantable murine reticulum sarcoma originating in ovary of C57BL/6 mice and highly invasive and metastatic[1-3]. When M5076 ovarian sarcoma is s.c. transplanted onto the backs of mice, solid tumor arises, spontaneously metastasizes to the liver and lung, and then kills the mice within about 25-30 days. This sarcoma exhibited lower sensitivity to antitumor agent as doxorubicin (DOX). Namely, M5076 ovarian sarcoma which has high metastasis and resistance, induced unfavorable prognosis on host body. In current chemotherapy, it is important for treatment on the sarcoma of these profiles.

Biochemical modulation is that the pharmacodynamics of the antitumor agent (effector) is modulated by combination with another drug (modulator) in order to enhance the antitumor activity, and the efficacy of chemotherapy is thereby enhanced. These studies have been performed extensively [4-10], and the enhancements of the activity of antitumor agents, e.g., 5-fluorouracil [6,7], are confirmed in clinical treatments. In this concept, there are two mechanisms for the increase in antitumor agent induced antitumor activity caused by a combined drug. The first mechanism, such as those involving UFT drugs (tegafur + uracil), constitutes the inhibition of the intracellular metabolism of antitumor agents, which leads to an increase in antitumor activity [4-7]. In the case of this mechanism, the modulator is specific to the antitumor agent. Namely, the modulator does not exhibit efficacy as with other antitumor agents. The second mechanism constitutes a change in the drug transport across the cell membrane, which leads to an increase in antitumor activity through elevation of the antitumor agent concentration in the tumor [8-10]. In the case of this mechanism, as these modulators act on the cell membrane transport of antitumor agents, the modulator may exhibit efficacy as with other antitumor agents, which are transported via the same transport processes.

When the modulators induced the enhancement of antitumor activities, there are some cases of increase in antitumor agent induced adverse reaction, in particular that by modulators in first mechanism. In this modulation, it appears to be not improved therapeutic index. Thus, the development of a novel modulator, which enhances antitumor activity and reduced adverse reactions of antitumor agents, has been needed. In addition, the use of modulators increases the number of medications and adds to the patient's burden. Simultaneously, the study to improve QOL of patients is also necessary. Meals were important at QOL of the patients in cancer chemotherapy. If the intake of food or beverage as modulator enhances efficacy of antitumor agent, then the improved antitumor activity by this type of biochemical modulation will reduce the patient's burden.

In this review point, I propose to be utilization of some food components in cancer chemotherapy on M5076 ovarian sarcoma, to improve cancer chemotherapy and to increase in QOL.

2. Theanine

2.1. Antitumor Activity

Many studies about biochemical modulation were not performed in the past in consideration of both the antitumor effects and adverse reactions of a drug, whereas green tea can be an ideal biochemical modulator because it has beneficial effects on both antitumor activity and adverse reactions of antitumor agent. As green tea is a common beverage, the combination of drinking green tea with chemotherapy is easy to try for human in clinical treatment.

The combination of theanine as specific amino acid in green tea, with DOX as antitumor agent was tried. In resistant tumors, the resistant is reversed by known drug combination-induced suppression on overexpressed P-glycoprotein and multidrug resistant associated protein, etc, with the inhibition of antitumor agent efflux from the resistant tumor cells. However, on the overexpression of these efflux pumps in normal tissues, these drug combinations also increase the adverse reaction of antitumor agent. Namely, these drug combinations do not induce an increase in the therapeutic index. We thought that the reversal of the drug resistance would be achievable by the common drug efflux pump for the resistance, and the effect of theanine on DOX permeability in P388 leukemia (P388) and DOX resistant P388 leukemia (P388/DOX) cells were examined. The effects of theanine on DOX efflux from P388 and P388/DOX cells are shown in Table 1. At 120 min after DOX efflux the efflux ratio of DOX in the P388 group was only 28% of that at 0 min, whereas this ratio in the P388/DOX group was 78%. In both cell lines DOX and theanine combined inhibited DOX efflux by 30.1% in P388 and 13.1% in P388/DOX cells. In contrast, the combination of verapamil, as P-glycoprotein inhibitor, with DOX inhibited DOX efflux by 59% in P388/DOX cells.

Next, the effect of the combined theanine on DOX induced antitumor activity was examined. In P388 cell bearing mice, DOX significantly decreased the tumor weight and theanine increased the DOX induced efficacy through an increase in the DOX concentration in the tumors (Table 2). Namely, the DOX concentration in the tumors in the DOX and theanine combined group were 1.5 fold of that in the DOX alone group in P388 bearing mice. On the other hand, in P388/DOX bearing mice, the DOX concentration in the tumor was 38 % of the level in the P388 tumor, and there was no change in the tumor weight on DOX only treatment. The combination of theanine with

DOX increased the DOX concentration in the tumor to the same level as in the P388 tumor, leading to significant antitumor activity. The increased DOX concentration in the tumor of P388 cell bearing mice after the combined DOX and theanine administration was the same as that in P388/DOX cell bearing mice. Therefore, these results suggested that theanine attacked the same transport process for DOX in both types of cells, elevated the DOX concentration and increased the DOX induced antitumor activity. Furthermore, it appears to be able to reverse the drug resistance through its efficacy on the common transport system in sensitive and resistant cells. In contrast, combined theanine did not affect DOX concentration in normal tissues, such as the heart and liver.

Table 1. Effects of theanine on DOX efflux from P388 and P388/DOX cells[a]

	P388	P388/DOX
0 min	2.579 ± 0.161	1.037 ± 0.058
120 min DOX alone	1.857 ± 0.101	0.282 ± 0.036
120 min DOX + theanine	2.074 ± 0.126	0.381 ± 0.062
	DOX + verapamil	0.728 ± 0.040
Inhibitory ratio with theanine(%)	30.1	13.1[b]

[a] DOX concentration in leukemia cells: $\mu g/10^7$ cells. [b] $P<0.05$: a significant difference from the DOX alone group level.

Table 2. Effect of theanine on the change of tumor weight induced by DOX

	Tumor weight (g)[a]	weight (g)[a]
	P388	P388/DOX
Control	1.76 ± 0.26[b]	0.60 ± 0.13
DOX alone	0.93 ± 0.19	0.52 ± 0.18
DOX + theanine	0.65 ± 0.21[c]	0.17 ± 0.06[b]

[a] Each value is the mean ± SD of eight mice. Significant differences from the level of DOX alone group are indicated by [b] $P < 0.001$ and [c] $P < 0.01$.

2.2. Antitumor Activity on Liver Metastasis

To advanced therapy on the intractable tumor, the effect of theanine on M5076 ovarian sarcoma cells [1-3], which has low sensitivity to DOX, was examined. The inhibitory effect on M5076 tumor growth was not observed by the administration of DOX alone (Figure 1). In contrast, the combination of theanine, as well as green tea, with DOX significantly decreased the tumor weight to 36 % of control level. Thus, these results demonstrate that theanine enhanced the antitumor activity of DOX against low sensitive tumor such as M5076 ovarian sarcoma, too. On the M5076 ovarian sarcoma, against which DOX was not effective, an antitumor effect of DOX was observed with the addition of theanine, without elevating the dose of DOX. Therefore, we may expect similar enhancement of antitumor activity by theanine against of low sensitivity tumor. These results suggest that theanine or green tea has a very important effect on cancer chemotherapy.

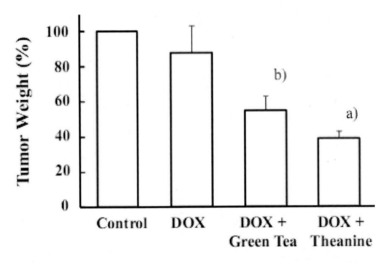

Figure 1. Effect of theanine on the changes in tumor weight (M5076) induced by DOX Each column is the mean ± SD of eight mice expressed as percentage of control level. Significant differences from the level of the DOX alone group are indicated by a) $P < 0.001$ and b) $P < 0.01$.

M5076 ovarian sarcoma is high metastasis tumor to the liver and lung. On M5076 ovarian sarcoma bearing mice in the condition of hepatic metastasis, the action of theanine on the inhibition of this metastasis induced by DOX was examined. On observation of the livers, the hepatic metastasis was graded, as to the metastasis area ratio in the liver, into five stages: metastasis score, 1 to 5. An increase in number of metastasis colonies was accompanied by an increase in liver weight. The liver is speculated to expand because of the hepatic metastasis of M5076. At that time, the relation coefficiency between the metastasis score and the relative liver weight (% liver/body weight) was $r^2 = 0.807$. Thus, the relative liver weight was demonstrated to be an indicator of hepatic metastasis. The normal liver comprises about 5 % of the body weight. In contrast with this, the relative liver weight of control mice transplanted with M5076 ovarian sarcoma significantly increased, and metastasis area occupied > 70% of the liver. In the DOX alone or DOX + theanine injected groups, the relative liver weights were decreased due to inhibition of hepatic metastasis. As shown in Figure 2, the metastasis scores were decreased in DOX group compared with that in the control group; furthermore, the combination with theanine significantly enhanced the metastasis suppressive efficacy of DOX. Thus, theanine amplified the suppressive efficacy of DOX on hepatic metastasis. Modulators that enhance the antitumor activity of chemotherapeutic agents against primary tumors and which are also effective in inhibiting subsequent metastasis have not be reported to date. Therefore, theanine was found to be a novel biochemical modulator, which enhances both the antitumor activity on primary tumor and also the inhibition of metastasis induced by antitumor agents. When M5076 was s.c. transplanted onto mice, in all cases, the M5076 metastasized to the liver within 20 days after tumor inoculation [1-3]. At the start of this treatment, tumor metastatic nodules were observed in the livers of all M5076 tumor bearing mice. Because the injection of DOX + theanine decreased the hepatic metastasis, it is suggested that DOX inhibited the growth of metastatic tumor in the liver, and then theanine enhanced the antitumor activity of DOX. In metastasized tumor, theanine presumably increases the DOX concentration; thus, effective antitumor activity of DOX against metastasis is obtained. Furthermore, during the treatment, tumor cells or minute colonies moved via blood vessels from the primary tumor to the metastatic area. When DOX was injected into mice followed by theanine, DOX was taken up by the tumor cells or colonies, and then theanine inhibited the release of DOX and increased the DOX accumulation in tumor colonies moving via blood vessels. Thus, it is expected that metastatic tumors circulating in vessels are killed by DOX with theanine before they reach the metastatic site. Consequently, the combined drug injection suppressed subsequent metastasis during the treatment. The inhibition of metastasis by the combination of theanine with DOX was possibly reflected by the reduction in primary tumor weight. However, the finding that pirarubicin, an anthracycline antibiotic, does not inhibit the hepatic metastasis of M5076, although pirarubicin significantly reduces the primary tumor weight [11], suggested that the inhibitory effect against primary tumor does not necessarily involve a suppression of metastasis. From another point of view, because theanine alone has never been found to inhibit tumor metastasis, it is suggested that theanine does not act on some metastatic mechanisms, such as adhesion and invasion. Therefore, theanine was demonstrated to enhance the DOX activity.

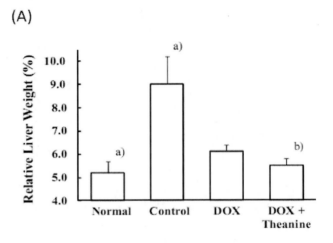

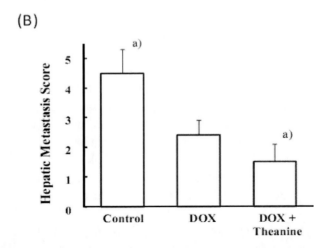

Figure 2. Effect of combined theanine on the relative liver weight (A) and hepatic metastasis (B) induced by DOX The relative liver weight is expressed as % (liver/body weight). The hepatic metastasis was graded, as to the metastasis area ratio in the liver, into five stages: metastasis score, 1 to 5. Each column represents the mean ± SD of eight mice expressed. Significant differences from the level of the DOX alone group are indicated by a) $P < 0.001$ and b) $P < 0.01$.

Namely, theanine was demonstrated to enhance the inhibition of hepatic metastasis induced by DOX due to increasing the DOX concentration in tumor cells. As theanine reduces the DOX concentration in the normal liver, theanine appears to increase the DOX concentration only in the hepatic metastasized tumor, i.e., not in normal liver. The transport mechanisms of some anthracycline derivatives in tumor cells were reported to be partly different from those in normal cells [12]. Judging from this evidence, it is possible that theanine acts on tumor in a different manner on normal tissues. With theanine, DOX was accumulated selectively in both primary and metastatic tumors, and the effective antitumor activity of DOX is obtained.

2.3. Glutamate Transporter

On the mechanism of the increase of DOX induced antitumor activity by theanine, the relation of glutamate transporters to theanine have been clarified. Theanine, a derivative of glutamate, enhanced the antitumor efficacy of DOX due to inhibition of the efflux of DOX from tumor cells.

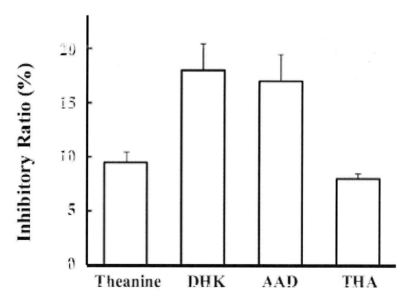

Figure 3. Effect of theanine and glutamate transporter inhibitors on the DOX efflux from M5076 ovarian sarcoma cells Each column represents the inhibitory ratio of DOX efflux (mean ± SD of four samples). Inhibitory ratio was calculated as (DOX efflux level for 120 min in the test drugs group/that the control group) x 100.

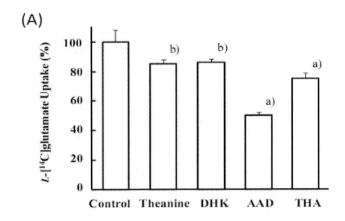

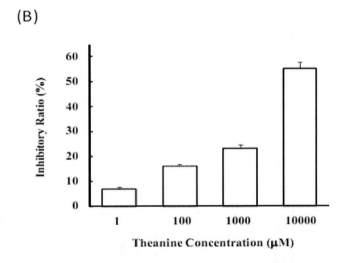

Figure 4. Effects of theanine (A: 100uM, B:1-10000uM) and glutamate transporter inhibitors on the L-(^{14}C)glutamate uptake by M5076 ovarian sarcoma cells. Each column represents the L-(^{14}C)glutamate uptake expressed as % of the control (mean ± SD of four samples). Significant differences from the control level are indicated by a) $P < 0.001$ and b) $P < 0.01$.

The effects of glutamate transport inhibitors, i.e. dihydrokinate (DHK), L-α-aminoadipate (AAD) and D,L-threo-β-hydroxyaspartate (THA), on the DOX efflux were examined in M5076 cells. As well as theanine, these inhibitors reduced the efflux of DOX (Figure 3), but did not change the influx of DOX. DHK, AAD and THA are structural analogues of glutamate, and competitively inhibit the uptake of glutamate and related substances [13]. However, the effects on the membrane transport of other drugs have never been reported to date. The fact that these glutamate analogues changed DOX efflux suggested that glutamate transporters should be related to the membrane transport of DOX in M5076 cells.

Furthermore, on glutamate uptake activity in M5076 cells, theanine, as well as glutamate transport inhibitors, DHK, AAD and THA, significantly reduced the glutamate uptake by 15% (Figure 4A). Moreover, theanine inhibited the glutamate uptake in a concentration-dependent manner (Figure 4B). Thus, theanine reduced the glutamate uptake similarly to the specific inhibitors. Since theanine was taken up by M5076 cells, it is expected that theanine was transported via glutamate transporters into M5076 cells and also competitively inhibited the glutamate uptake. The inhibition of DOX efflux by glutamate transport inhibitors suggested that theanine inhibits the DOX efflux with a reduction of glutamate uptake.

Five types of glutamate transporter were cloned, and their tissue distributions and physiological functions were investigated [14-18]. Some of them were shown to be expressed in tumor cells, such as C6 glioma and hepatoma cells [18-20]. In the examination of expressing glutamate transporters (four subtypes, GLT-1, GLAST, EAAC1 and EAAT4) in M5076 cells by RT-PCR analysis. GLAST and GLT-1 were detected in M5076 cells. Moreover, Western blot analysis expected the expression of GLAST and GLT-1 in M5076 cells. From the results, these two subtypes were estimated to bring glutamate into M5076 cells. As regards, the affinity of inhibitors to glutamate transporter subtypes, EAAC1 was reported to be more sensitive to AAD than to DHK [13,15]. In contrast, GLT-1 was sensitive to both DHK and AAD, and GLAST was most sensitive to THA among the three inhibitors [13,21]. According to these physiological properties, the expression of GLAST and GLT-1 in M5076 cells corresponds to the inhibition of glutamate uptake by the inhibitors.

GLAST and GLT-1, astrocytic glutamate transporters, are abundantly expressed mostly in the cerebellum and telencephalon, respectively (18). These high affinity glutamate transporters terminate the transmission by removing glutamate from the synaptic cleft and prevent neuronal damage from excessive activation of glutamate receptors [22,23]. The inhibition of glutamate transporters increases the extracellular glutamate concentration and excessive accumulation of glutamate causes neuronal death. In GLAST mutant mice, it has been reported that inhibition of GLAST enhanced glutamate neurotoxicity and increased the susceptibility to cerebellar injury [24].

Similarly, homozygous mice deficient in GLT-1 were shown to induce lethal spontaneous epileptic seizures and increased susceptibility to acute cortical injury [25]. Inhibiting glutamate uptake, theanine may possibly enhance the toxicity of glutamate. However, the reduction of glutamate uptake by theanine was weaker than that by the specific inhibitors DHK, AAD and THA. Although theanine is distributed in brain tissues [26], its toxicity has never been reported to date. On the other hand, DOX can not permeate through the blood-brain barrier and, therefore, is not distributed in brain tissues. Therefore, the combination of DOX and theanine are not likely to cause neurotoxicity. Theanine was reported to be an antagonist of the N-methyl-Daspartate (NMDA) receptor, one of the glutamate receptors related to the neuronal death induced by glutamate [26]. Accordingly, theanine could protect brain tissues from glutamate neurotoxicity.

Since DOX and theanine exhibit no similarity in chemical structure, it is probably impossible for DOX to be transported directly across glutamate transporters. The process of efflux of DOX by tumor cells could not be explained only by this membrane transport.

It is speculated that the decrease in the concentration of glutamate in tumor cells caused by theanine induced a change in the intracellular level of glutathione (GSH). It has also been suggested that the level of GSH in tumor cells is connected with drug sensitivity and that a decrease in the intracellular level of GSH induced an enhancement of drug sensitivity [27]. Furthermore, a GS-X pump, which transports the GSH conjugate of a drug, has been identified. It has been suggested that the GS-X pump causes the release of antitumor agents in tumor cells and is connected with multidrug resistance [28,29]. As well as buthionine sulfoximine (BSO) [30], a specific inhibitor of γ-glutamylcystenyl-synthetase (γ-GCS), the rate-limiting enzyme for GSH, theanine significantly decreases the intracellular concentration of GSH in M5076 cells, to 78% of the normal level (Figure 5). Namely, the inhibition of glutamate uptake by theanine was considered to induce a decrease in the synthesis of GSH from glutamate as a substrate. It has been reported that suppression of the intracellular uptake of glutamate in glutamate-free medium induced a decrease in the intracellular level of GSH [31], which was supported by these results. The decrease in GSH evoked with the combination of theanine and DOX was shown to be greater than that caused by DOX alone. Furthermore, the amount of GS-DOX conjugate in the presence of theanine decreased to 85% of that in the DOX alone group (Figure 5). Namely, the intracellular generation of the GS-DOX conjugate was confirmed to decrease with the theanine induced reduction in the level of GSH.

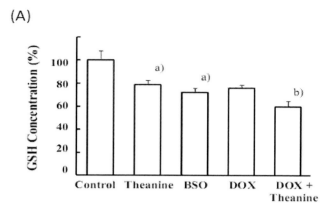

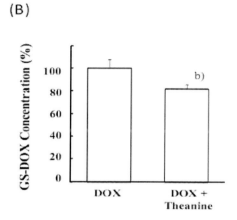

Figure 5. Effect of theanine on the glutathione (A) and doxorubicin-glutathione conjugate (B) concentrations in M5076 ovarian sarcoma cells. M5076 cells were incubated with theanine or BSO (100 μ M), or DOX (9.0 nmol/ml). GSH concentrations are expressed as% of the control level (mean $\pm$ S.D., $n=4$). GS-DOX concentrations are expressed as % of the level in the DOX alone group (mean $\pm$ S.D., $n=4$). A significant difference from the control level is indicated by (a) $P < 0.001$. A significant difference from the level for the DOX alone group is indicated by (b) $P < 0.05$.

The GS-X pump, which is responsible for the extracellular transport of the GSH conjugate, appears to be a member of the ABC transporter family [31,32]. Multidrug resistance associated protein (MRP) was reported to transport the GSH conjugate ATP-dependently and to be a code for the GS-X pump. Namely, MRP family members eliminate the GSH conjugate as a transport substance and compose a detoxification system for xenobiotics in the cell. In M5076 cells, the expression of MRP5, which functions in the efflux of DOX, was confirmed. We speculated that the GS-DOX conjugate was transported extracellularly via the MRP5/GS-X pump in M5076 cells.

It has been suggested that the MRP/GS-X pump, which differs from P-glycoprotein that functions as a drug transport pump without any help, is closely connected with the intracellular metabolic system for GSH [29]. The conjugated reaction between GSH and drugs is catalyzed by a glutahione S-transferase (GST). In particular, GST-π is closely related to the drug sensitivity of tumor cells and the level of GST-π is reported to be correlated with drug efflux [34]. Like theanine, BSO, as an inhibitor of γ-GCS, and ketoprofen, as an inhibitor of GST-π, significantly suppressed the efflux of DOX from M5076 cells. Therefore, it is considered that the GSH biosynthetic and conjugative reactions are closely connected with the efflux of intracellular DOX and that the efflux decreases with the inhibition of these reactions.

From these results, we speculated on the mechanism for the theanine induced effect, as follows. Some of the DOX taken up by M5076 cells binds to GSH and thereby generates the GS-DOX conjugate. The conjugate is released extracellularly by the M5076/GS-X pump. This pathway is closely connected with the intracellular synthesis of GSH and the GSH conjugated reaction, which was supported by the finding that the efflux of DOX was suppressed by BSO and ketoprofen. On the other hand, theanine suppressed the uptake of glutamate and thereafter the biosynthesis of GSH through inhibition of GLAST and GLT-1 as glutamate transporters in M5076 cells. Then, generation of the conjugate of intracellular DOX and GSH is affected and the release of the GS-DOX conjugate by tumor cells via the MRP5/GS-X pump decreases. It is considered that these phenomena suppress the decrease in the concentration of DOX in a tumor and induce the increase in the DOX induced antitumor activity caused by theanine. As GLAST and GLT-1 are not expressed in the heart and liver, theanine did not have an effect in these tissues. In the brain, where GLAST and GLT-1 are expressed, DOX is not present. Thus, we concluded that the combination of theanine with DOX is an ideal chemotherapy for increasing antitumor activity without intensifying adverse reaction.

Theanine is an amino acid existing in green tea, and sufficient intake of theanine can be achieved by daily drinking of green tea. Furthermore, theanine appears to have less toxicity than conventional chemotherapeutic agents. Namely, concerning safety cancer chemotherapy theanine is more useful than medicine.

3. Anserine

Anserine is a dipeptide, consisting of L-histidine and alanine, and is contained in the skeletal muscles of fowl and migratory fish (cf: 980 mg/100 g chicken). The details of the pharmacological effects of anserine are not clear. However, anserine has been applied as a supplement due to its antioxidative effect [34,35].

Using M5076 ovarian sarcoma bearing mice, there was no change in tumor size and tumor weight as a result of DOX treatment. In contrast, the combination of anserine with DOX significantly decreased the tumor size and tumor weight. It was considered that anserine increased DOX induced antitumor activity by the maintenance of the DOX concentration in the tumor, as the DOX concentration in the tumor in the anserine + DOX group was 1.5-fold that in the DOX alone group. On the other hand, anserine has no effect on DOX concentration in normal tissues. It is expected that anserine does not increase the DOX induced adverse reaction, rather it decreases by antioxidative effect of anserine [34,35]. Thus, anserine appeared to increase the antitumor activity of DOX with increasing the DOX concentration in the tumor by the specific action on the tumor.

Furthermore, anserine significantly induced DOX influx compared with that in the DOX alone group, whereas it did not change the level of DOX efflux. Namely, it is speculated that the mechanism by which anserine induced an increase of the antitumor activity by DOX was due to the promotion of the DOX influx into tumor cells. Anserine consists of histidine and alanine whereas there was no effect on the DOX influx by both amino acids. Thus, it has been clarified that anserine was shown to act in the DOX induced antitumor activity as the mother compound, not after metabolism. The combined L-valine-methylester or glycyl-sarcosine (as the inhibitor of dipeptide transporter) with anserine suppressed the effect of anserine on the DOX influx. Namely, it was speculated that anserine was taken into tumor cells via dipeptide transporter and exhibited the increase of the DOX influx. Furthermore, anserine did not have the effect on DOX metabolism.

4. Taurine

Taurine is an aminosulfonic acid, which comprises 1-2% in seafood, including top shell, cuttlefish, and sea plum. Taurine has been used as a medicine to improve hepatic function in congested heart failure and hyperbilirubinemia. Taurine has a regulatory effect on calcium in cardiac muscle, lowers blood pressure, and increases the excretion of bile acid. Taurine is widely used as a supplement to help recovery from stress.

Taurine significantly inhibited DOX efflux, which resulted in the once of maintain DOX levels in M5076 cells. *In vivo* experiments, taurine administration decreased tumor weight by 40%, compared to the DOX-alone group and significantly increased its antitumor effect.

Taurine transport is changed osmotic pressure in cell. Namely, these changes by taurine were considered to induce the changes of other transporters on DOX transport in tumor cells. Taurine is transported by a taurine transporter (TAUT), but it was not indicated that TAUT are connected with the membrane transport of DOX. The TAUT belongs to the SLC6A6 family, which contains various nerve transmitter substances, has over ten subtypes. Taurine is recognized as a substrate of the TAUT, and β-alanine are TAUT inhibitors. The chemical structure of these inhibitors is similar to that of taurine and they are competitive substrates. β-alanine and taurine are β- amino acids, and have high affinity for TAUT. TAUT may contribute to taurine uptake in keratinocyte. There are not a report on the expression of SLC6A6 transporter in M5076 ovarian sarcoma cells. However, the intracellular uptake of [^{3}H]-taurine was confirmed. β-alanine inhibited [^{3}H]-taurine accumulation by 77.7% ($P<0.001$) and by 31.3% ($P <0.001$) at 3 and 10 min, respectively, compared to the control level. Thus, it is speculated that TAUT expresses in a M5076 tumor cell membrane. β-alanine acts only as a taurine transporter inhibitor, and it is not a substrate of other transport systems. Namely, it was considered that the uptake of DOX was prevented by a decrease in cellular uptake of taurine via the effect of β-alanine as a taurine transporter inhibitor. As DOX influx was inhibited by β-alanine, which acts only on the taurine transporter and taurine enhanced the DOX level, enhancement of the DOX level by taurine addition was suggested to act via taurine transport.

5. Cucuribitacin E

cucurbitacin E provides the bitter taste to thesquash family and is classified as a triterpenoid derivative (36). Cucurbitacin derivatives have antihepatotoxic and anti-inflammatory effects that are mediated by pharmacological inhibition of COX-2. In DOX permeability in M5076 cells,

SAM

7/7/14

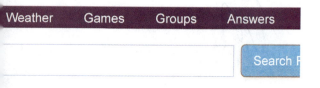

our guaranteed sources of income, like Social
guaranteed income must come from your savi

ing you take the desired withdrawals, and see
, but assume you spend $5,000 more or less a
all changes in your spending can make the dif

estment goal in retirement is not to maximize
rincipal. What most retirees want is sustainabl

cucurbitacin E promoted of DOX influx and suppressed DOX efflux. These effects appeared when using a low concentration of cucurbitacin E (10 nM). For this time course in influx system, the effects of cucurbitacin E appeared in the late stages of incubation, thus the action mechanism of cucurbitacin E was likely related DOX efflux. In the DOX influx system, DOX was taken into tumor cells at an early time and released from at later time points. In the early stages of incubation, the DOX concentration in tumor cells was lower than that in the medium and the simple diffusion rate was influx > efflux. In contrast, the DOX concentration in tumor cells at later time points was increased, and the rate was influx < efflux. It is therefore likely that the inhibitory effect of cucurbitacin E on DOX efflux also affected DOX influx, resulting in apparent promotion of DOX influx by cucurbitacin E.

In vivo, DOX treatment did not change in the time course of tumor size and tumor weight in M5076 ovarian sarcoma, compared to control levels. In contrast, the combination of cucurbitacin E with DOX was decreased tumor size and tumor weight, compared to that in DOX alone group, indicating effective antitumor activity. The combined cucurbitacin E treatment showed a tendency for decreased DOX levels in normal tissues, compared to that of DOX only group. In particular, DOX level in the heart was significantly decreased by the combined treatment with cucurbitacin E, suggesting that cucurbitacin E may decrease DOX-induced cardiotoxicity. In contrast, the combination of cucurbitacin E with DOX did not change DOX levels in the tumor. Based on the reduction of tumor size and tumor weight, combined treatment with cucurbitacin E appeared to increase the DOX-induced antitumor activity in vivo. Furthermore, cucurbitacin E application was shown to sustain DOX concentration in tumor cells in vitro. We originally hypothesized that cucurbitacin E induced increases in DOX activity were caused by increased DOX concentration in the tumor. However, the intratumorial DOX concentrations were similar between the DOX alone group and DOX + cucurbitacin E group at 48 h after treatment. On the other hand, the DOX concentration in the tumors in M5076 ovarian sarcoma-bearing mice at 8 h after DOX administration increased significantly by combined cucurbitacin E. Thus, the DOX level in simultaneous treatment with DOX and cucurbitacin E was shown to be 9.2-fold higher ($P < 0.05$) than the DOX alone level, and the level in the post treatment of cucurbitacin E group was 4.5-fold higher than the DOX alone level. In contrast, the DOX concentration in normal tissues showed a tendency to decrease with cucurbitacin E treatment. It was expected that the different effects of cucurbitacin E between the tumor and normal tissues was a result of differences in the expression of transporters in the cell membranes of tumor cells and normal cells. In the transport system of DOX efflux in M5076 ovarian sarcoma cells, GS-DOX conjugate was produced by the binding of DOX and glutathione (GSH), which was then transported by the MRP/GS-X pump complex [27,37]. The overexpression of MRP5 was confirmed in M5076 ovarian sarcoma cell membranes [38,39]. MRP is expressed in many normal tissues and is comprised of MRP1-MRP9 as members of the MRP family [40]. The expression of MRP subfamily members is known to differ in tumor cells and other tissues [41]. Namely, the different effects of cucurbitacin E between the tumor and normal tissues were speculated to be a result of differences in the MRP subtypes. The cucurbitacin E-enhanced antitumor activity of DOX was suggested to be related to the increased concentration of DOX in the tumor shortly after cucurbitacin E administration.

In conclusion, it was suggested that the suppression of DOX efflux by cucurbitacin E in vitro induced an increase in DOX concentration in the tumor, which increased the DOX antitumor activity. Furthermore, it was speculated that the attack point of cucurbitacin E was an MRP. The combination of cucurbitacin E with DOX may therefore be an effective tool with broad applications in cancer chemotherapy.

Conclusion

On M5076 ovarian sarcoma cells, theanine and taurine as amino acid, anserine as dipeptide, and cucurbitacin E enhanced antitumor activity of DOX. In conclusion, it is expected that the combination of food components with antitumor agent advances novel therapy on some sarcomas.

References

[1] Talmadge, J. E., Key, M. E., and Hart, I. R. Characterization of amurine ovarian reticulum cell sarcoma of histiocytic origin. *Cancer Res.*, 41: 1271–1280, 1981.

[2] Talmadge, J. E., and Hart, I. R. Morphologic studies on a murine reticulum cell sarcoma (histiocytic sarcoma) of histiocytic origin and its metastasis. *Vet. Pathol.*, 20: 342–352, 1983.

[3] Hart, I. R., Talmadge, J. E., and Fidler, I. J. Metastatic behavior ofa murine reticulum cell sarcoma exhibiting organ-specific growth. *Cancer Res.*, 41: 1281–1287, 1981.

[4] Konishi, T., and Dezuki, Y. Biochemical modulation. *CRC Crit. Rev.*, 1: 88-97, 1992.

[5] Hidalgo, O. F., Gonzalez, F., Gil, A., Campbell, W., Barrajon, E. and Lacave, A. J. 120 hours simultaneous infusion of cisplatin and fluorouracil in metastatic breast cancer. *Am. J. Clin. Oncol.*, 12: 397-401, 1989.

[6] Bertino, J. R., Sawicki, W. L., Lindquist, C. A., and Gupta, V. S.Schedule dependent antitumor effects of methotrexate and 5-fluorouracil. *Cancer Res.*, 37: 327-328, 1977.

[7] Bud, G. 1., Fleming, R. M., Bukowski, R. M., McCracken, J. D., and Rinvkin, S. E. 5-Fluorouracil and folinic acid in the treatment of advanced coborectal cancer: a randomized comparison. A Southwest Oncology Group Study. *J. Clin. Oncol.*, 5: 272-277, 1987.

[8] Sadzuka, Y., Iwazaki, A., Miyagishima, A., Nozawa, Y., and Hirota, S. Effects of methybxanthine derivatives on Adriamycin concentration and antitumor activity. *Jpn. J. Cancer Res.*, 86: 594-599, 1995.

[9] Sadzuka, Y., Sugiyama, T., Miyagishima, A., Nozawa, Y., and Hirota, S. The effects of theanine, as a novel biochemical modulator, on the antitumor activity of Adriamycin. *Cancer Lets.*, 105: 203-209, 1996.

[10] Sadzuka, Y., Sugiyama, T., and Hirota, S. Modulation of cancer chemotherapy by green tea. *Clin. Cancer Res.*, 4: 153–156, 1998.

[11] Sugiyama, T., Sadzuka, Y., Miyagishima, A., Nozawa, Y., Nagasawa, K., Ohnishi, N., and Yokoyama, T. Membrane transport on tumor cell and antitumor activity of doxorubicin and pirarubicin. *Drug Delivery System*, 13: 35–40, 1998.

[12] Nagasawa, K., Ohnishi, N., and Yokoyama, T. Transport mechanisms of idarubicin, an anthracycline derivative, in human leukemia HL60 cells and mononuclear cells, and comparison with those of its analogs. *Jpn. J. Cancer Res.*, 88: 750–759, 1997.

[13] Kanai, Y., Smith, C. P., and Hediger, M. A. A new family of transmitter transporters: the high-affinity glutamate transporters. *FASEB J.*, 7: 1450–1459, 1993.

[14] Sugiyama, T., and Sadzuka, Y. Enhancing effects of green tea components on the antitumor activity of adriamycin against M5076 ovarian sarcoma, *Cancer Lett.* 133: 19–26, 1998.

[15] Kanani, Y., and Hediger, M.A. Primary structure and characterization of a high-affinity glutamate transporter. *Nature* 360: 467–471,1992.
[16] Storck, T., Schulte, S., Hofmann, K., and Stoffel, W. Structure, expression and functional analysis of a Na+-dependent glutamate/aspartate transporter from rat brain. *Proc. Natl. Acad. Sci. USA* 89: 10955–10959, 1992.
[17] Pines, G., Danbolt, N.C., Bjoras, M., Zhang, Y., Bendahan, A., Eide, L., Koepsell, H., Storm-Mathisen, J., Seeberg, E., and Kanner, B.I. Cloning and expression of a rat brain L-glutamate transporter. *Nature* 360: 464–467, 1992.
[18] Gegelashvili, G., and Schousboe, A. Cellular distribution and kinetic properties of high-affinity glutamate transporters. *Brain Res. Bull.* 45: 233–238, 1998.
[19] Dowd, L.A., Coyle, A.J., Rothstein, J.D., Pritchett, D.B., and Robinson, M.B., Comparison of Na+-dependent glutamate transport activity in synaptosomes, C6 glioma, and Xenopus oocytes expressing excitatory amino acid carrier 1 (EAAC1). *Mol. Pharmacol.* 49: 465–473, 1993.
[20] McGivan, J.D., Rat hepatoma cells express novel transporter systems for glutamine and glutamate in addition to those present in normal rat hepatocytes. *Biochem. J.* 330: 255–260, 1998.
[21] Klockner, U., Storck, T., Conradt, M., Stoffel, W. Functional properties and substrate specificity of the cloned L-glutamate/L-aspartate transporter GLAST-1 from rat brain expressed in Xenopus oocytes. *J. Neurosci.* 14: 5759–5765, 1994.
[22] Nicholls, D., and Attwell, D. The release and uptake of excitatory amino acids. *Trends Neurosci.* 11: 462–468, 1990.
[23] Watkins, J.C. and Evans, R.H., 1981. Excitatory amino acid transmitters. *Annu. Rev. Pharmacol. Toxicol.* 21: 165–204, 1981.
[24] Watase, K., Hashimoto, K., Kano, M., Yamada, K., Watanabe, M., Inoue, Y., Okuyama, S., Sakagawa, T., Ogawa, S., Kawashima, N., Hori, S., Takimoto, M., Wada, K., and Tanaka, K. Motor discoordination and increased susceptibility to cerebellar injury in GLAST mutant mice. *Eur. J. Neurosci.* 10: 976–988, 1998.
[25] Tanaka, K., Watase, K., Manabe, T., Yamada, K., Watanabe, M., Takahashi, K., Iwama, H., Nishikawa, T., Ichihara, N., Kikuchi, T., Okuyama, S., Kawashima, N., Hori, S., Takimoto, M., and Wada, K. Epilepsy and exacerbation of brain injury in mice lacking the glutamate transporter GLT-1. *Science* 276: 1699–1702, 1997.

[26] Yokogoshi, H., Kobayashi, M., Mochizuki, M., and Terashima, T. Effect of theanine, -glutamylethylamide, on brain monoamines and striatal dopamine release in conscious rats. *Neurochem. Res.* 25: 667–673, 1998.
[27] Zhang, K., Yang, E.B., Wong, K.P., and Mack, P. GSH, GSH-related enzymes and GS-X pump in relation to sensitivity of human tumor cell lines to chlorambucil and adriamycin. *Int. J. Oncol.* 14: 861–867, 1999.
[28] Ishikawa, T. The ATP-dependent glutathione S-conjugate export pump. *Trends Biochem. Sci.* 17: 463–468, 1992.
[29] Ishikawa, T., Wright, C.D., and Ishizuka, H., GS-X pump is functionally overexpressed in cis-diamminedichloro-platinum(II)-resistant human leukemia HL-60 cells and downregulated by cell differentiation. *J. Biol. Chem.* 269: 29085–29093, 1994.
[30] Griffith, O.W., and Meister, A. Potent and specific inhibition of glutathione synthesis by buthionine sulfoximine(S-n-butyl homocysteine sulfoximine). *J. Biol. Chem.* 254: 7558–7560, 1979.
[31] Reichelt, W., Stabel-Burow, J., Pannicke, T., Weichert, H., and Heinemann, U. The glutathione level of retinal muller glial cells is dependent on the high-affinity sodium dependent uptake of glutamate. *Neuroscience* 77: 1213–1224, 1997.
[32] Ishikawa, T. The GS-X pump family: ATP dependent multispecific organic anion transporters. *Protein. Nucleic Acid, Enzyme* 42: 1285–1294, 1997.
[33] Niitu, Y., Ishigaki, S., Takahashi, Y., Hirata, Y., Saito, T., Arisato, N., Hosoda, K., Watanabe, and N., Hohgo, Y. GST-assay For Serodiagnosis of Malignancy. *Glutathione S-transferase and Drug Resistance*. Taylor Francis, London, pp. 409–417, 1990.
[34] Young, S., Kwon, H.Y., Kwon, O.B., and Kang, J.H., Hydrogen peroxide-mediated Cu, Zn–superoxide dismutase fragmentation: protection by carnosine, homocarnosine and anserine. *Biochim. Biophys. Acta* 1472: 651–657, 1999.
[35] Kang, J.H., Kim, K.S., Choi, S.Y., Kwon, H.Y., Won, M.H., and Kang, T.C. Protective effects of carnosine, homocarnosine and anserine against peroxyl radical-mediated Cu, Zn–superoxide dismutase modification. *Biochim. Biophys. Acta* 1570: 89–96, 2002.
[36] Jayaprakasam, B., Seeram, N.P., and Nair, M.G. Anticancer and anti-inflammatory activities of cucurbitacins from Cucurbita andreana. *Cancer Res.* 189: 11–16, 2003.
[37] Priebe, W., Krawczyk, M., Kuo, M.T., Yamane, Y., Savaraj, N., and Ishikawa, T. Doxorubicin- and daunorubicin- glutathione conjugates, but

not unconjugated drugs, competitively inhibit leukotriene C4 transport mediated by MRP/GS-X pump. *Biochem. Biophys Res. Commun.* 247: 859–863, 1998.

[38] Sadzuka, Y., Sugiyama, T., Tanaka, K., and Sonobe, T. Inhibition of glutamate transporter by theanine enhances the therapeutic efficacy of doxorubicin. *Toxicol. Lett.* 121: 89–96, 2001.

[39] Sadzuka, Y., Sugiyama, T., Suzuki, and Sonobe, T. Enhancement of the activity of doxorubicin by inhibition of glutamate transporter. *Toxicol. Lett.* 123: 159–167, 2001.

[40] Borst, P., Evers, R., Kool, M., and Wijnholds, J. The multidrug resistance protein family. *Biochim. Biophy. Acta* 1461: 347–357, 1999.

[41] Nooter, K., Westerman, A.M., Flens, M.J., Zaman, G.J.R., Scheper, R.J., van Wingerden, K.E., Burger, H., Oostrum, R., Boersma, T., Sonneveld, P., Gratama, J.W., Kok, T., Eggermont, A.M.M., Bosman, F.T., and Stoter, G. Expression of a multidrug resistance-associated protein (MRP) gene in human cancers. *Clin. Cancer Res.* 1: 1301–1310, 1995.

In: Sarcoma
Editor: Eric J. Butler

ISBN: 978-1-62100-362-5
© 2012 Nova Science Publishers, Inc.

Chapter IV

Advances in Chondrosarcoma Treatment: Engineering in vitro Three-Dimensional Models

YuLong Han[1,2], LiHong Zhou[1], ShuQi Wang[3], JinHui Wu[4], ZhenFeng Duan[5], TianJian Lu[1] and Feng Xu[1,2,3]**

[1]Biomedical Engineering and Biomechanics Center,
Xi'an Jiaotong University, Xi'an 710049, P.R. China
[2]School of Life Science and Technology,
Xi'an Jiaotong University, Xi'an 710049, P.R. China
[3]HST-Center for Biomedical Engineering, Department
of Medicine, Brigham and Women's Hospital,
Harvard Medical School, Boston, MA, U. S.
[4]State Key Laboratory of Pharmaceutical Biotechnology,
Nanjing University, Nanjing 210093, P.R. China
[5]Center for Sarcoma and Connective Tissue Oncology, Massachusetts
General Hospital, Harvard Medical School, MA, U. S.

---

*Corresponding authors: fxu2@rics.bwh.harvard.edu, tjlu@mail.xjtu.edu.cn.

1. Introduction

Chondrosarcoma is a common bone cancer that affects thousands of people worldwide. Although chondrosarcoma has been recognized for a long time, little breakthrough has been achieved in the treatment. Currently, surgery is the only effective treatment, despite the fact that it negatively affects the patient's life quality and has high risks of recurrence [1]. To address this, various treatment regimens based on radiotherapy and chemotherapy have been developed, which however showed limited success due to the cancer's resistance to radiotherapy and chemotherapy [2]. This clinical situation can be improved by further understanding on cancer-treatment interactions, which depends on the availability of clinically relevant *in vitro* models. However, existing cancer models are mainly based on two-dimensional (2D) culture, which has shown significantly different behaviors compared to native three-dimensional (3D) cancer tissues [3-6]. Emerging novel biomaterials (e.g., hydrogels) and tissue engineering methods offer great potential to address these challenges [7]. In this chapter, we present state-of-the-art advances in chondrosarcoma treatment and *in vitro* cancer models, with focus on engineering 3D cell microenvironment. These achievements may lead to the foundation of basic research and bridge the gap between lab research and clinical treatment.

2. Advances in the Clinical Treatment of Chondrosarcoma

2.2. Chondrosarcoma

Chondrosarcoma has various clinical presentations and morphologies and it is characterized by over production of chondrocytes and cartilage matrix [2].Chondrosarcoma is one of the primary malignantbone cancers [2, 8] and accounts for approximately 25% of bone cancer cases [9, 10]. Chonadrsarcoma can occur at any age with a preference in old people, approximately 62% of whom are diagnosed in their forties to sixties [11].Chondrosarcoma can originate from multiple body sites, where chondrosarcoma in trunk (e.g., pelvis, ribs and shoulder girdle) accounts for ~66% of all chondrosarcoma [11, 12]. Surgery is the first therapeutic choice for chondrosarcoma in clinics due to the resistance of chondrosarcoma to chemical and radiation therapies [13]. Despite radical surgical removal of cancer tissues, the 10-year survival rate for chondrosarcoma patients is still low, e.g., barely 29% for patients with grade III [14]. The management of chondrosarcoma is complicated in clinics due to limited available effective therapies and variable clinical presentations. For example, tumors may have different behaviors although they have a similar histopathologic appearance from a clinical point of view [15].

For better clinical management, chondrosarcoma is classified according to parameters, i.e., grade and subtype. Based on the cellularity, nuclear size, mitotic rate, and gravity, chondrosarcoma can be divided into grade I, II and III with poorer clinical outcome for higher grade. The grade of chondrosarcoma is strongly associated with death rate, metastasis rate, and recurrence rate [16] and thus has been used as a prognostic factor [17]. Alternatively, chondrosarcoma can be divided into five subtypes, including classical (conventional) chondrosarcoma, dedifferentiated chondrosarcoma, mesenchymal chondrosarcoma, clear cell chondrosarcoma, and periosteal (Juxtacortical) chondrosarcoma [18]. These subtypes are defined according to the histology of chondrosarcoma tissues (e.g., cell type, differentiation, matrix, architecture) and clinical presentations [19]. Classical chondrosarcoma

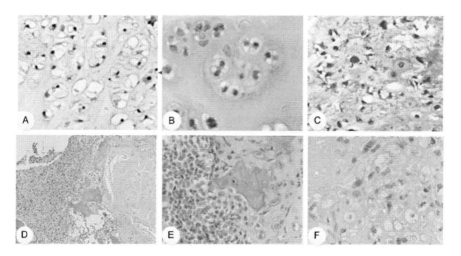

Figure 1. Histology of different chondrosarcoma subtypes [19, 111, 117, 118]. (A)-(C) Grade I, II and III chondrosarcoma, (D) Dedifferentiated chondrosarcoma, (E) Mesenchymal chondrosarcoma, (F) Clear cell chondrosarcoma.

accounts for 90% of all chondrosarcoma [19], and can be further divided into primary (central) chondrosarcoma and secondary (peripheral) chondrosarcoma according to their location in the bone [20]. Each of the five chondrosarcoma subtypes has its own histologic characteristics (Figure 1) [21].

2.3. Surgery

The goal of chondrosarcoma treatments is to minimize the risks of cancer recurrence, metastasis, and death without comprising the life quality of patients [1]. To this end, various therapeutic methods have been developed, including surgery, radiotherapy and chemotherapy.

Currently, surgery is the first therapeutic option of chondrosarcoma in clinics and adequate surgical excision remains to be the only efficient way [19]. The management of surgical resection varies according to different clinical presentations (e.g., location, subtype, size of neoplasm, grade). Surgical margin is a main factor relating to recurrence rate and morbidities [16, 22]. Generally, wide, en bloc excision (removal of all neoplasm and part of tissue around) is applicable to patients with high grade chondrosarcoma (grade II and higher)[17, 22]. Bone reconstruction is needed sometimes after wide excision depending on the tumor location (e.g., weight-bearing bones) [23]. However, not all the high-grade chondrosarcoma can be completely resected, especially chondrosarcoma in spine and pelvis. These unresected chondrosarcoma challenges all the existing clinical therapies, indicative of an urgent need for novel effective therapies. In contrast to high-grade chondrosarcoma, the preferred management of low-grade chondrosarcoma (grade I) is intralesional surgery (e.g., curettage) due to the low recurrence and metastasis potential [1]. However, the 'adequate surgical excision' is not well defined and the clinical management is still on debate[21].Although intralesional surgery and wide resection have no significant difference in view of cancer control (e.g., recurrence rate and death rate), intralesional surgery has better functional outcomes and less complications than wide resection[24]. For instance, positive outcomes have been reported on treating low-grade chondrosarcoma with combination of intralesional surgery and cryosurgery [25-27]. However, intralesional surgery has also been reported to cause increased recurrence rate compared to that in wide resection. It was reported that intralesional surgery for chondrosarcoma of pelvis was associated with100% of recurrence rate [28], indicating that the position of chondrosarcoma should also be taken into account. Besides, patients with intra-articular, radiographically aggressive or large size low-grade chondrosarcoma tend to have wide resection [21, 29].

In summary, to balance the life quality post-surgery and the control level of disease, wide resection is preferred for high grade and resectable chondrosarcoma while accumulating evidence indicates that intralesional surgery is preferred for low grade chondrosarcoma.

2.4. Radiotherapy

For patients with unresectable chondrosarcoma (*e.g.*, chondrosarcoma of skull and spine), radiotherapy is the main treatment to control cancer and alleviate symptoms [30, 31].However, chondrosarcoma is relatively radio-resistant, e.g., the dose required for local control is greater than 60Gy [32], which is comparable to the tolerant dose of surrounding normal tissue [1, 33]. To improve the effect of radiotherapy, many methods have been developed, such as introduction of protons and heavy ions instead of photons to form a more localized distribution of radiation within the tumor [34, 35].

Proton therapy has become a favorable treatment of chondrosarcoma because of controllable energy delivery along proton beam pathway and sharply energy reduction within a few millimeters, minimizing the damage of surrounding normal tissues [32, 36, 37]. For instance, the 5 year local control rate of unresectable chondrosarcoma ranges from 75~100% after treatment using particle therapies with proton or proton-photon [37].

Another type of particle that is promising for radiotherapy of chondrosarcoma is heavy ion such as carbon and the combination of helium and neon [21]. Particle therapies with carbon are attractive due to its controlled energy distribution and improved biological effectiveness [38]. The 5 year survival rate can reach 98.2% according to Daniela Schulz-Ertner's report [39]. Although carbon ion based therapies achieved excellent results, it is not yet proved to obtain better clinical outcomes than protons based therapies which are the gold standard for unresectable chondrosarcoma, due to the small size of the cohort study [34].

2.5. Chemotherapy

Although some researchers found that patients with certain chondrosarcoma (i.e., dedifferentiated chondrosarcoma and mesenchymal chondrosarcoma) benefited from chemotherapy, most chondrosarcoma (e.g., conventional chondrosarcoma) are chemoresistant [1]. Thus, there is no gold standard chemotherapy yet.

The effect of chemotherapies on dedifferentiated chondrosarcoma, a fatal disease with the worst prognosis [40, 41], is controversial. In an initial study, Mitchell et al. [42] reported an improved survival rate in patients. However, following studies showed that dedifferentiated chondrosarcoma poorly respond to chemotherapies [43, 44]. Most of these researches have a small size of cohort studies due to the rarity of chondrosarcoma patients, and retrospective study seems to be the only way to reach a statistic conclusion. According to some retrospective studies [45, 46], chemotherapies did not significantly affect the outcome in terms of the survival rate. Although beneficial results have also been reported for chemotherapies of mesenchymal chondrosarcoma [47, 48], it should be noted that small sample sized were used in these cohort studies.

Due to the rarity of both dedifferentiated chondrosarcoma and mesenchymal chondrosarcoma (less than 10% of all chondrosarcoma cases), the advance in the therapeutic and basic researches significantly limited. The emerging *in vitro* models that recapitulate native chondrosarcoma are promising to address this challenge.

2.6. Emerging New Therapies

Emerging therapies such as photodynamic therapy (PDT) and target treatment hold great potential to treat chondrosarcoma. PDT involves the administration of photosensitizer (or prephotosensitizer) within cancer tissues and subsequent irradiation of photosensitizer using a certain wavelength of light to kill cancer cells by inducing release of Reactive Oxygen Specis (ROS)[49]. PDT has been applied to induce chondrosarcoma necrosis since 1989 through damaging blood vessels around the tumor in a mouse model [50]. The clinical application of PDT in chondrosarcoma of hyoid is reported recently [51], in which a reduced tumor size was observed after treatment. These studies indicate that PDT may become a reliable tool in the management of chondrosarcoma because of low side-effects.

Compared to PDT, targeted therapies of chondrosarcoma have also been proposed with the advances in the understanding of chondrosarcoma biology [19, 52, 53]. These promising targets are schematically shown in Figure 2. However, most of these therapeutic targets are based on size-limited cohorts.

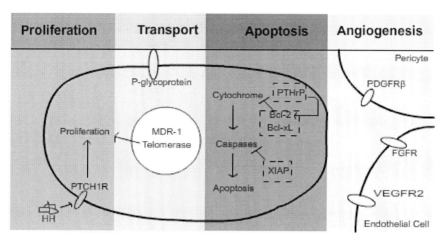

Figure 2. Therapic targets for chondrosarcoma. The targets of chondrosarcoma can be divided into four groups: proliferation, transport system, apoptosis and angiogenesis. IHH (Indian Hedge-hog) signaling is a significant pathway in the development of chondrocyte and has been found to regulate the proliferation of chondrosarcoma [112]. Upon this pathway, the Hedgehog (HH) is a main target and its antagonists such as Cyclopamine or Triparanol have been tested for clinical treatment. Besides, telomerase activity enhances the cell proliferation and can be inhibited by BIBR1532 [113]. G-glycoprotein, coded by MDR-1 gene, is responsible for the efflux-mediated drug resistance [114]. PTHrP, Bcl-2, Bcl-xL, and XIAP are related to the suppression of apoptosis [115, 116]. PDGFRβ, FGFR and VEGFR2 are the key receptors in angiogenesis and can be inhibited by SU6668 [80].

To confirm the applicability of targeted therapy in clinics, more studies with a relative large cohort are needed. Moreover, the signaling pathways in different chondrosarcoma subtypes may differ from each other, which necessitate further studies to identify subgroup specific targets [52]. However, target therapies face the same challenges as chemotherapies due to the low incidence of chondrosarcoma. Tissue engineering may provide a niche to study the biological mechanism of chondrosarcoma and provide a platform to screen for effective treatment methods. This requires the joint efforts from clinicians, biologists and engineers.

3. *In vitro* Models of Chondrosarcoma

3.1. In vitro Cancer Models

Various cancer models have been developed in vitro for basic cancer research and clinical studies [54]. Most of these models are based on 2D cultures (e.g., culture on surface of flasks, cover slips) due to their easy availability [55]. Although significant advances have been made on our understanding of cancer behaviors (e.g., genetics [56]), these 2D culture models are associated with several limitations as compared to 3D or in vivo situations. For instance, the spatial gradient distribution of oxygen and nutrition in the native tumor anatomic structure is missing in 2D model, which affect cell biology significantly [57].

Tumor cells grow in a complicated 3D microenvironment that is composed of various extracellular matrix (ECM) components and cell types [58], which are positioned in 3D with specific spatial distribution. The microenvironment components play an important role in almost every aspect of cancer behavior, e.g., the interaction between lung epithelium cells and chondrosarcoma increase its invasiveness [13]. However, these important factors of cancer microenvironment are missing in most 2D culture models [5, 6], which may partially explain the situation of limited breakthroughs in cancer treatment over the past 10 years [59].

Accumulating evidence demonstrates that cancer cells in 3D models behave differently from those in 2D models, such as metabolism [60], gene-expression [61], and drug sensitivity [62]. For instance, cancer cells in 3D models respond differently (including sensitizing and desensitizing) from 2D models when exposed to drugs [63]. Besides, some cancer cells do not grow well in the conventional culture system. For example, prostate cell lines (e.g., LNCaP series) have limited adhesion to conventional dishes [64] and chordoma cells showed difficulties when cultured in current conventional culture system [65]. 3D models may better recapitulate in vivo cancer response to chemotherapeutic treatment [66]. Therefore, 3D cancer models hold great potential to address these challenges by bridging in vitro and in vivo situations.

Various chondrosarcoma cell lines have been used to develop in vitro models to study the biology of chondrosarcoma and to screen for effective drugs. However, the existing cell lines cannot represent the heterogeneous group as observed in clinics (clinical presentations). Despite the limitation, cell lines covering all subtypes and grades with different origin sites are needed in the basic research to engineer 3D models and set up animal models.

3.2. Animal Models of Chondrosarcoma

Animal models have played a significant role in chondrosarcoma study (e.g., signal pathway, therapy assessment) [67].One of the most predominant chondrosarcoma animal models is Swarm rat chondrosarcoma (SRC) [68-70]. This well-established model is histologically and phenotypically stable in that SRC cells are well-differentiated and type II collagen is secreted [71], which provides a good in vivo platform to study chondrosarcoma. The SRC initially originated from a Sprague-Dawley rat, and the diseased tissue was isolated and then transplanted into other rats [68]. During the transplantation, swarm rat chondrosarcoma lost its ability to produce bone elements and became a real chondrosarcoma producing cartilage elements only [69, 72]. To improve the clinical relevance of this model, however, orthotropic transplantation, namely injection of tumor cells into intramedullary canal instead of subcutaneous tissue, is necessary [73]. However, the clinical relevance is significantly limited by the original subtype of this tumor in current derived SRC animal models.

Another popular chondrosarcoma animal model is nude mice transplanted with different human chondrosarcoma cell lines [74, 75]. Compared to allograft (e.g., SRC), xenograft (e.g., nude mice) of human original tumor is more useful to study the biology of human chondrosarcoma and assess potential therapeutic strategies. Of all xenogrfat models, nude mice are prominent in clinical relevance because of immune incompetence. Otherwise, administration of immune suppressants would be required, which can affect cancer biology [76]. Up to now, various nude mice models have been developed based on chondrosarcoma several cell lines including OUMS-27 [77], HCS-2/A [74], NCDS-1 [78], HCS-TG [79], and SW1353 [80].

Although animal models can better mimic native tumor tissues compared to *in vitro* 2D culture, the disadvantages are obvious. The cost of animal models is high and using animal models leads to a long experiment cycle. Allograft (i.e., Swarmt rat) has poor clinical relevance, whereas xenograft (i.e., nude mice) suffers from missing immune cells which play an important role in tumor biology [81]. In addition, the use of animal models requires ethical approval, which may be an issue in certain countries.

4. Engineering 3D Microenvironment of Chondrosarcoma

4.1. Microenvironment of Chondrosarcoma *in vivo* and Its Effect on Biology

Significant social and financial efforts have been made on cancer research since the declaration of the war against cancer by American president Nixon in 1971. However, statistics do not show any decline of mortality caused by cancers [82]. The 'soil and seed' hypothesis proposed by Paget one hundred years ago draw public attention again, which indicates that the cell microenvironment (soil) affect the cancer metastasis significantly [83]. Recently, more and more evidence supports this point and shows that microenvironment of cancer can affect tumor behaviors such as tumorigenesis, tumor growth and metastasis [81, 82, 84-88]. However, the microenvironment differs from one tumor to another, it is necessary to review the effects of microenvironment on the biological behavior of chondrosarcoma.

Microenvironment of caner is a complicate system including surrounding cells and extracellular matrix [82], which interacts with tumor cells physically and chemically. For chondrosarcoma, the effects of microenvironment have been extensively studied in Swarm rat models [89], where transplantation of chondrosarcoma into different sites (i.e., subcutaneous and tibia) resulted in different tumor phenotypes. The chondrosarcoma in subcutaneous grows faster than that in tibia according to the average tumor weight after 3-week transplantation (35.05g versus 75.22mg). It is also found that chondrosarcoma in tibia behaved more aggressively, causing bone destruction and secondary lung colonization. These findings from animal test confirm that that cell microenvironment affects the physiology and anatomy of chondrosarcoma. In human neoplasm, microenvironmental parameters, such as hypoxia, can affect chondrosarcoma behaviors including angiogenesis [90], malignancy [91, 92] and invasiveness [93].

Compared with molecular mechanism such as P-glycoprotein, microenvironmental factors are believed to contribute more to intrinsic drug resistance of chondrosarcoma. ECM acts as a native barrier to drug diffusion. As characterized by the WHO, chondrosarcoma is a cancer disease with overproduction of cartilage-specific ECM. The diseased cartilage tissue is low vascularized and this further reduces the accessibility of drug molecules. Hypoxia is also associated with under vascularization in tumor tissue and it enhances the poor tissue perfusion and causes slow growth [94], thus resulting in resistance to the targeted treatment. Cell-cell interaction and cell-ECM interaction promote the multidrug resistance by E-cadherin and integrin, respectively [95-97].To our knowledge, this kind of multiple drug resistance has not been investigated in chondrosarcoma.

Accumulating evidence has proven that the microenvironment of chondrosarcoma contributes to its biology and drug resistance [98]. For instance, the remote cells like lung epithelium also induce metastasis of chondrosarcoma to lung by secreting stromal cell-derived factor I [13]. However, most of the environmental factors observed *in vivo* are missing in the basic research of chondrosarcoma as well as drug screening *in vitro*. The tissue engineering approach is a promising way to recapitulate chondrosarcoma *in vitro*, Figure 3.

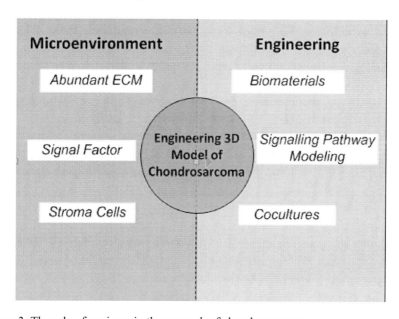

Figure 3. The role of engineer in the research of chondrosarcoma.

4.2. Methods for Engineering 3DCancer Cell Microenvironment

The milestone study of 3D cancer models was performed by Bissell *et al.* on the integrin blocking transform malignant phenotype into nonmalignant phenotype [99]. This study indicated that cell-ECM interactions played a prominent role in tumor cell behavior. Currently, 3D cancer models can be divided into two categories [55]: encapsulating cells into porous biomaterials and enhancing the formation of tumor spheroids in suspension. The applications of these models require a convenient method to fabricate these 3D models in a high throughput manner, e.g., for high throughput drug screening. In order to mimic native tumor, the *in vitro* model should include main factors such as cell-stroma, cell-cell, and cell-ECM interactions. Here, we present some emerging methods that are promising to investigate chondrosarcoma *in vitro*.

Cancer spheroids have been generated as *in vitro* disease models and candidates for drug screening. Conventional methods include spinner flask culture [100] and rotary wall vessel reactor [101]. These spheroids partly mimic the environments of tumor including tumor cell-cell interaction and the gradient of nutrition. To reduce complexity in constructing those 3D cancer models by these methods, microwell array has been developed and used for cancer drug screening due to the high throughput capability and controllable cell microenvironment [102, 103].

In contrast, encapsulating cells in biomaterials (e.g., hydrogels) is a promising approach due to the controllable 3D cell microenvironment [104]. Basically, cells are suspended in hydrogel precursor solution, which is then gelled (e.g., through micromolding, photolithography, or bioprinting) to provide cells a 3D microenvironment. Different biomaterials have been developed to encapsulated cells, including natural materials and synthetic materials. Matrigel is one of the most widely used natural hydrogels and holds great potential to mimic the environment of chondrosarcoma. Matrigel is a basement membrane commercialized available, which is derived from a rat chondrosarcoma [55] and contains abundant various molecules (e.g., ECM proteins, signal factors [105]), which can be used to modulate cell behaviors. With the support of Matrigel in 3D, cancer cells form spheroids. These spheroids can recapitulate the cell-cell interaction between and cell-ECM interaction. However, the main challenge associated with Matrigel is that its components are not well defined and batch-to-batch variations are commonly observed [105]. Compared with natural materials, synthetic materials have gained the popularity in recent years due to its modifiable biochemical and biophysical properties [106, 107]. For example, PEG and its derivatives comprise a main part of synthetic materials due to the perfect biocompatibility and easy control of polymerization [108]. Further, cell printing is rapidly developed to fabricate complex tissue structures [109]. This system has recently been used to investigate the cell-cell interaction in an ovarian cancer research [110].

5. Conclusions and Prospects

Chondrosarcoma is a highly malignant cancer with various clinical presentations and intrinsic resistance to chemo- and radio- therapies. Deeper understanding on the mechanism of treatment resistance is essential to develop new therapies at the cellular level, which has been lacking over the past 30 years. Recent studies have shown that the microenvironment that chondrosarcoma resides in plays a significant role in chondrosarcoma biology and its resistance to chemo- and radio- therapies. A significant challenge to study chondrosarcoma is low incidence of clinical cases specially the rare subtypes, and the limited availability of reliable *in vitro* models. Although various 2D models have been developed, these models lack some important *in vivo* microenvironmental factors. The emerging tissue engineering approaches such as encapsulating cells in 3D hydrogels offer a niche to investigate the interactions between microenvironment and cancer cells in 3D models. These approaches hold great potential to engineer the 3D microenvironment of chondrosarcoma *in vitro*, and provide a reliable cancer model to explore new therapies. The success of this strategy needs further efforts and collaboration from different areas, including engineering, biology, and medicine.

References

[1] Riedel, R., et al., The clinical management of chondrosarcoma. *Current Treatment Options in Oncology*, 2009. 10(1): p. 94-106.

[2] Onishi, A., A. Hincker, and F. Lee, Surmounting chemotherapy and radioresistance in chondrosarcoma: molecular mechanisms and therapeutic targets. *Sarcoma*, 2011. 2011: p. 381564.

[3] Rizvi, I., et al. *Biologically relevant 3D tumor arrays: treatment response and the importance of stromal partners*. 2011. San Francisco, California, USA: SPIE.

[4] Hakanson, M., M. Textor, and M. Charnley, Engineered 3D environments to elucidate the effect of environmental parameters on

drug response in cancer. *Integrative Biology (Camb)*, 2011. 3(1): p. 31-8.

[5] Yamada, K.M. and E. Cukierman, Modeling tissue morphogenesis and cancer in 3D. *Cell,* 2007. 130(4): p. 601-10.

[6] Fischbach, C., et al., Engineering tumors with 3D scaffolds. *Nature Methods,* 2007. 4(10): p. 855-60.

[7] Geckil, H., et al., Engineering hydrogels as extracellular matrix mimics. *Nanomedicine* (Lond), 2010. 5(3): p. 469-84.

[8] A. L. Hartley, V.B., M. Harris, J. M. Birch, S. S. Banerjee, A. J. Freemont, J. McClure, and L. J. McWilliam, Sarcomas in north west England: II. Incidence. *British Journal of Cancer*, 1991. 64(6): p. 1145–1150.

[9] Spjut. H. J.. Dorfman, H.D., Fechner, R. E., and Ackerman, L. V. , ed. *Tumors of bone and cartilage.* 1971, Armed Forces Institute of Pathology.: Washington, DC. 84-116.

[10] Pathology., o., ed. Tumors and tumor-like lesions of the bone.*Pathology, radiology and treatment*, 1994, Springer-Verlag: Berlin. 201-256.

[11] Zenmyo, M., et al., Gadd45ß expression in chondrosarcoma: a pilot study for diagnostic and biological implications in histological grading. *Diagnostic Pathology,* 2010. 5: p. 69.

[12] Pant, R., et al., Chondrosarcoma of the scapula. *Cancer,* 2005. 104(1): p. 149-158.

[13] Lai, T.-H., et al., Stromal cell-derived factor-1 increase αvβ3 integrin expression and invasion in human chondrosarcoma cells. *Journal of Cellular Physiology,* 2009. 218(2): p. 334-342.

[14] Schrage, Y.M., et al., Kinome profiling of chondrosarcoma reveals Src-Pathway activity and dasatinib as option for treatment. *Cancer Research,* 2009. 69(15): p. 6216-6222.

[15] Dahlin, D.C. and E.D. Henderson, Chondrosarcoma, A surgical and pathological problem: review of 212 cases. *Journal of Bone Joint Surgery(American Volume).,* 1956. 38(5): p. 1025-1125.

[16] Evans, H.L., A.G. Ayala, and M.M. Romsdahl, Prognostic factors in chondrosarcoma of bone. A clinicopathologic analysis with emphasis on histologic grading. *Cancer,* 1977. 40(2): p. 818-831.

[17] LEE, F.Y., et al., Chondrosarcoma of Bone: An Assessment of Outcome. *Journal of Bone Joint Surgery(American Volume)*, 1999. 81(3): p. 326-38.

[18] F.Schajowicz, ed. *Histological typing of bone tumours.* Second Edition ed., ed. L.H.Sobin. 1993, Springer: Heidelberg.

[19] Bovée, J.V.M.G., et al., Emerging pathways in the development of chondrosarcoma of bone and implications for targeted treatment. *The Lancet Oncology*, 2005. 6(8): p. 599-607.
[20] Bertoni F, B.P., Hogendoorn PCW, Pathology and genetics of tumours of soft tissue and bone. *World Health Organisation classification of tumours.* 2002, Lyon: IARC Press.
[21] Gelderblom, H., et al., The clinical approach towards chondrosarcoma. *Oncologist*, 2008. 13(3): p. 320-329.
[22] F. Fiorenza, A.A., R. J. Grimer, S. R. Carter, R. M. Tillman, K. Ayoub, D. C. Mangham, A. M. Davies, Risk factors for survival and local control in chondrosarcoma of bone. *The Journal of Bone and Joint Surgery(British Volume)*, 2002. 84-B(93-9).
[23] Moran, S.L., A.Y. Shin, and A.T. Bishop, The use of massive bone allograft with intramedullary free fibular flap for limb salvage in a pediatric and adolescent population. *Plastic and Reconstructive Surgery*, 2006. 118(2): p. 413-419 10.1097/01.prs.0000227682.71527.2b.
[24] Aarons, C., et al., Extended intralesional treatment versus resection of low-grade chondrosarcomas. *Clinical Orthopaedics and Related Research®*, 2009. 467(8): p. 2105-2111.
[25] Hanna, S.A., et al., Outcome of intralesional curettage for low-grade chondrosarcoma of long bones. *European Journal of Surgical Oncology (EJSO)*, 2009. 35(12): p. 1343-1347.
[26] Veth, R., et al., Cryosurgery in aggressive, benign, and low-grade malignant bone tumours. *The Lancet Onco*logy, 2005. 6(1): p. 25-34.
[27] Mohler, D., et al., Curettage and cryosurgery for low-grade cartilage tumors is associated with low recurrence and high function. *Clinical Orthopaedics and Related Research®*, 2010. 468(10): p. 2765-2773.
[28] Streitbürger, A., et al., Grade I chondrosarcoma of bone: the Münster experience. *Journal of Cancer Research and Clinical Oncology*, 2009. 135(4): p. 543-550.
[29] Leerapun, T., et al., Surgical management of conventional grade I chondrosarcoma of long bones. *Clinical Orthopaedics and Related Research*, 2007. 463: p. 166-172 10.1097/BLO.0b013e318146830f.
[30] Tzortzidis, F., et al., Patient outcome at long-term follow-up after aggressive microsurgical resection of cranial base chondrosarcomas. *Neurosurgery*, 2006. 58(6): p. 1090-1098 10.1227/01.NEU.0000215892.65663.54.
[31] Almefty, K., et al., Chordoma and chondrosarcoma: Similar, but quite different, skull base tumors. *Cancer*, 2007. 110(11): p. 2467-2477.

[32] Noël, G., et al., Radiation therapy for chordoma and chondrosarcoma of the skull base and the cervical spine. *Strahlentherapie und Onkologie,* 2003. 179(4): p. 241-248.

[33] Habrand, J.L., et al., Neurovisual outcome following proton radiation therapy. *International Journal of Radiation Oncology*Biology*Physics,* 1989. 16(6): p. 1601-1606.

[34] Nikoghosyan, A., et al., Randomised trial of proton vs. carbon ion radiation therapy in patients with low and intermediate grade chondrosarcoma of the skull base, clinical phase III study. *BMC Cancer,* 2010. 10(1): p. 606.

[35] Nguyen, Q.-N. and E. Chang, Emerging role of proton beam radiation therapy for chordoma and chondrosarcoma of the skull base. *Current Oncology Reports,* 2008. 10(4): p. 338-343.

[36] Peeters, A., et al., How costly is particle therapy? Cost analysis of external beam radiotherapy with carbon-ions, protons and photons. *Radiotherapy and Oncology,* 2010. 95(1): p. 45-53.

[37] Amichetti, M., et al., A systematic review of proton therapy in the treatment of chondrosarcoma of the skull base. *Neurosurgical Review,* 2010. 33(2): p. 155-165.

[38] Tsujii, H., et al., Overview of clinical experiences on carbon ion radiotherapy at NIRS. *Radiotherapy and Oncology,* 2004. 73(Supplement 2): p. S41-S49.

[39] Schulz-Ertner, D., et al., Carbon ion radiotherapy of skull base chondrosarcomas. *International Journal of Radiation Oncology*Biology*Physics,* 2007. 67(1): p. 171-177.

[40] Bruns, J., et al., Dedifferentiated chondrosarcoma—a fatal disease. *Journal of Cancer Research and Clinical Oncology,* 2005. 131(6): p. 333-339.

[41] Sopta, J., et al., Dedifferentiated chondrosarcoma: our clinico-pathological experience and dilemmas in 25 cases. *Journal of Cancer Research and Clinical Oncology,* 2008. 134(2): p. 147-152.

[42] Mitchell, A.D., et al., Experience in the treatment of dedifferentiated chondrosarcoma. *J. Bone Joint Surg. Br.,* 2000. 82-B(1): p. 55-61.

[43] Dickey, I.D., et al., Dedifferentiated chondrosarcoma: the role of chemotherapy with updated outcomes. Journal of Bone and Joint Surgery*(American Volume),* 2004. 86(11): p. 2412-2418.

[44] Dickey, I.D., et al., Dedifferentiated chondrosarcoma: the role of chemotherapy. *Journal of Bone and Joint Surgery (British Volume),* 2008. 90-B(SUPP_I): p. 114-.

[45] Staals, E.L., P. Bacchini, and F. Bertoni, Dedifferentiated central chondrosarcoma. *Cancer*, 2006. 106(12): p. 2682-2691.
[46] Grimer, R.J., et al., Dedifferentiated chondrosarcoma: Prognostic factors and outcome from a European group. *European Journal of Cancer*, 2007. 43(14): p. 2060-2065.
[47] Marilena Cesari, F.B., Patrizia Bacchini, Mario Mercuri, Emanuela Palmerini, Stefano Ferrari, Mesenchymal chondrosarcoma. An analysis of patients treated at asingle institution. *Tumori*, 2007. 93: p. 4.
[48] Dantonello, T.M., et al., Mesenchymal chondrosarcoma of soft tissues and bone in children, adolescents, and young adults. *Cancer*, 2008. 112(11): p. 2424-2431.
[49] Plaetzer, K., et al., Photophysics and photochemistry of photodynamic therapy: fundamental aspects. *Lasers in Medical Science*, 2009. 24(2): p. 259-268.
[50] Reed MW, M.A., Anderson GL, Miller FN, Wieman TJ., The effect of photodynamic therapy on tumore oxygenation. *Surgery*, 1989. 106(1)(94-9).
[51] Nhembe, F., et al., Chondrosarcoma of the hyoid treated with interstitial photodynamic therapy. Head andamp; *Neck Oncology*, 2009. 1(0): p. 1-1.
[52] Bovée, J.V.M.G., et al., Cartilage tumours and bone development: molecular pathology and possible therapeutic targets. *Nature Reviews Cancer*, 2010. 10(7): p. 481-488.
[53] Papachristou, D.J. and A.G. Papavassiliou, Osteosarcoma and chondrosarcoma: New signaling pathways as targets for novel therapeutic interventions. *The International Journal of Biochemistry and Cell Biology*, 2007. 39(5): p. 857-862.
[54] Sharma, S.V., D.A. Haber, and J. Settleman, Cell line-based platforms to evaluate the therapeutic efficacy of candidate anticancer agents. *Nature Reviews Cancer*, 2010. 10(4): p. 241-53.
[55] Lee, J., M.J. Cuddihy, and N.A. Kotov, Three-dimensional cell culture matrices: state of the art. *Tissue Engineering Part B: Reviews*, 2008. 14(1): p. 61-86.
[56] Balmain, A., Cancer genetics: from Boveri and Mendel to microarrays. *Nature Reviews Cancer*, 2001. 1(1): p. 77-82.
[57] Gabriel Helmlinger, F.Y., Marc Dellian and Rakesh K. Jain, Interstitial pH and pO2 gradients in solid tumors in vivo: High-resolution measurements reveal a lack of correlation. *Nature Medicine*, 1997. 3: p. 5.

[58] Bissell, M.J. and D. Radisky, Putting tumours in context. *Nature Reviews Cancer,* 2001. 1(1): p. 46-54.
[59] Hutmacher, D.W., Biomaterials offer cancer research the third dimension. *Nature Materials,* 2010. 9(2): p. 90-93.
[60] Evenou, F., T. Fujii, and Y. Sakai, Spontaneous formation of highly functional three-dimensional multilayer from human hepatoma Hep G2 cells cultured on an oxygen-permeable polydimethylsiloxane membrane. *Tissue Engineering Part C: Methods,* 2010. 16(2): p. 311-318.
[61] Feder-Mengus, C., et al., New dimensions in tumor immunology: what does 3D culture reveal? *Trends in Molecular Medicine,* 2008. 14(8): p. 333-340.
[62] Loessner, D., et al., Biomaterials bioengineered 3D platform to explore celle-ECM interactions and drug resistance of epithelial ovarian cancer cells. *Biomaterials,* 2010. 31(32): p. 8494-8506.
[63] Serebriiskii, I., et al., Fibroblast-derived 3D matrix differentially regulates the growth and drug-responsiveness of human cancer cells. *Matrix Biology,* 2008. 27(6): p. 573-585.
[64] Gurski, L.A., et al., Hyaluronic acid-based hydrogels as 3D matrices for in vitro evaluation of chemotherapeutic drugs using poorly adherent prostate cancer cells. *Biomaterials,* 2009. 30(30): p. 6076-6085.
[65] Lucia Ricci-Vitiani, P.D., Francesco Pierconti, M.D., P.D. Maria Laura Falchetti, Giovanna Petrucci, Ph.D., Giulio Maira, M.D., And M.D. Ruggero De Maria, Luigi Maria Larocca, M.D., And Roberto Pallini, M.D., Establishing tumor cell lines from aggressive telomerase-positive chordomas of the skull base. *Journal of Neurosurgery,* 2006.
[66] Farach-Carson, L.A.G.N.J.P.X.J.a.M.C., 3D matrices for anti-cancer drug testing and development. *Oncology Issues,* January 2010.
[67] Clark, J.C.M., C.R. Dass, and P.F.M. Choong, Development of chondrosarcoma animal models for assessment of adjuvant therapy. *ANZ Journal of Surgery,* 2009. 79(5): p. 327-336.
[68] Maibenco, H.C., R.H. Krehbiel, and D. Nelson, Transplantable osteogenic tumor in the rat. *Cancer Research,* 1967. 27(2 Part 1): p. 362-366.
[69] Breitkreutz, D., et al., Histological and biochemical studies of a transplantable rat chondrosarcoma. *Cancer Research,* 1979. 39(12): p. 5093-5100.
[70] Dissertations, C.H.-T.a., *Functional genomic analyses of the impact of global hypomethylation and of tumor microenvironment in a rat model of human chondrosarcoma.* 2009.

[71] Stevens, J.W., Heterogeneity in growth properties of the rat wwarm chondrosarcoma. *Iowa Orthop. J.* , 2004. 24: p. 33-35.
[72] Choi, H.U., K. Meyer, and R. Swarm, Mucopolysaccharide and Protein—Polysaccharide of a transplantable rat chondrosarcoma. *Proceedings of the National Academy of Sciences*, 1971. 68(5): p. 877-879.
[73] Grimaud E, D.C., Rousselle AV, Passuti N, Heymann D, Gouin F., Bone remodelling and tumour grade modifications induced by interactions between bone and swarm rat chondrosarcoma. *Histology and Histopathology,* 2002. 17: p. 1103-11.
[74] Takigawa, M., et al., Establishment from a human chondrosarcoma of a new immortal cell line with high tumorigenicity in vivo, which is able to form proteoglycan-rich cartilage-like nodules and to respond to insulin in vitro. *International Journal of Cancer*, 1991. 48(5): p. 717-725.
[75] Schrage, Y.M., et al., COX-2 expression in chondrosarcoma: A role for celecoxib treatment? *European journal of cancer* (Oxford, England : 1990), 2010. 46(3): p. 616-624.
[76] Luan, F.L., et al., Rapamycin blocks tumor progression: unlinking immunosuppression from antitumor efficacy1. *Transplantation*, 2002. 73(10): p. 1565-1572.
[77] Kunisada, T., et al., A new human chondrosarcoma cell line (OUMS-27) that maintains chondrocytic differentiation. *International Journal of Cancer,* 1998. 77(6): p. 854-859.
[78] Kudo, N., et al., Establishment of novel human dedifferentiated chondrosarcoma cell line with osteoblastic differentiation. *Virchows Archiv.,* 2007. 451(3): p. 691-699.
[79] Kudawara, I., et al., New cell lines with chondrocytic phenotypes from human chondrosarcoma. *Virchows Archiv.*, 2004. 444(6): p. 577-586.
[80] Frank M Klenke, A.A., Elisabeth Bertl, Martha-Maria Gebhard, Volker Ewerbeck, Peter E uber, Axel Sckell, Tyrosine kinase inhibitor SU6668 represses chondrosarcoma growth via antiangiogenesis in vivo. B*MC Cancer,* 2007. 7(49).
[81] Yu, H., M. Kortylewski, and D. Pardoll, Crosstalk between cancer and immune cells: role of STAT3 in the tumour microenvironment. *Nature Reviews Immunology,* 2007. 7(1): p. 41-51.
[82] Albini, A. and M.B. Sporn, The tumour microenvironment as a target for chemoprevention. *Nature Reviews Cancer*, 2007. 7(2): p. 139-147.
[83] Paget, S., The distribution of secondary growths in cancer of the breast.*The Lancet*, 1889. 133(3421): p. 571-573.

[84] Mueller, M.M. and N.E. Fusenig, Friends or foes [mdash] bipolar effects of the tumour stroma in cancer. *Nature Reviews Cancer,* 2004. 4(11): p. 839-849.

[85] Bierie, B. and H.L. Moses, Tumour microenvironment: TGF[beta]: the molecular Jekyll and Hyde of cancer. *Nature Reviews Cancer,* 2006. 6(7): p. 506-520.

[86] Måseide, K., T. Kalliomäki, and R. Hill, Microenvironmental effects on tumour progression and metastasis, in *integration/interaction of oncologic growth*, G. Meadows, Editor. 2005, Springer Netherlands. p. 1-22.

[87] Liotta, L.A. and E.C. Kohn, The microenvironment of the tumour-host interface. *Nature,* 2001. 411(6835): p. 375-379.

[88] Finger, E. and A. Giaccia, Hypoxia, inflammation, and the tumor microenvironment in metastatic disease. *Cancer and Metastasis Reviews,* 2010. 29(2): p. 285-293.

[89] Hamm, C., et al., Microenvironment alters epigenetic and gene expression profiles in Swarm rat chondrosarcoma tumors. *BMC Cancer,* 2010. 10: p. 471.

[90] Kubo, T., et al., Expression of hypoxia-inducible factor-1{alpha} and its relationship to tumour angiogenesis and cell proliferation in cartilage tumours. *The Journal of Bone and Joint Surgery(British Volume),* 2008. 90-B(3): p. 364-370.

[91] Lin, C., et al., Hypoxia induces HIF-1α and VEGF expression in chondrosarcoma cells and chondrocytes. *Journal of Orthopaedic Research,* 2004. 22(6): p. 1175-1181.

[92] Boeuf, S., et al., Correlation of hypoxic signalling to histological grade and outcome in cartilage tumours. *Histopathology,* 2010. 56(5): p. 641-651.

[93] Sun, X., et al., CXCR4/SDF1 mediate hypoxia induced chondrosarcoma cell invasion through ERK signaling and increased MMP1 expression. *Molecular Cancer,* 2010. 9: p. 17.

[94] Fallica, B., G. Makin, and M.H. Zaman, Bioengineering approaches to study multidrug resistance in tumor cells. *Integrative Biology,* 2011. 3(5): p. 529-539.

[95] Dalton, W.S., The tumor microenvironment as a determinant of drug response and resistance. *Drug resistance updates,* 1999. 2(5): p. 285-288.

[96] Green, S.K., et al., Antiadhesive antibodies targeting E-cadherin sensitize multicellular tumor spheroids to chemotherapy in vitro. *Molecular Cancer Therapeutics*, 2004. 3(2): p. 149-159.
[97] Wu, R.C., et al., ß2-integrins mediate a novel form of chemoresistance in cycloheximide-induced U937 apoptosis. *Cellular and Molecular Life Sciences*, 2004. 61(16): p. 2071-2082.
[98] E. David, F.B., M. F. Heymann, G. De Pinieux, F. Gouin, F. Rédini, D. Heymann, The bone niche of chondrosarcoma: A sanctuary for drug resistance, tumour growth and slso a source of new therapeutic targets. *Sarcoma*, 2011.
[99] Weaver, V.M., et al., Reversion of the malignant phenotype of human breast cells in three-dimensional culture and in vivo by integrin blocking antibodies. *The Journal of Cell Biology*, 1997. 137(1): p. 231-245.
[100] Sutherland, R.M., et al., A multi-component radiation survival curve using an in vitro tumour model. International Journal of Radiation Biology, 1970. 18(5): p. 491-495.
[101] Lin, R.-Z. and H.-Y. Chang, Recent advances in three-dimensional multicellular spheroid culture for biomedical research. *Biotechnology Journal*, 2008. 3(9-10): p. 1172-1184.
[102] Hakanson, M., M. Textor, and M. Charnley, Engineered 3D environments to elucidate the effect of environmental parameters on drug response in cancer. *Integrative Biology*, 2011. 3(1): p. 31-38.
[103] Hardelauf, H., et al., Microarrays for the scalable production of metabolically relevant tumour spheroids: a tool for modulating chemosensitivity traits. *Lab. on a Chip*, 2011. 11(3): p. 419-428.
[104] Burdett, E., et al., Engineering tumors: atissue engineering perspective in cancer biology. *Tissue Engineering Part B: Reviews*, 2010. 16(3): p. 351-359.
[105] Kleinman, H.K. and G.R. Martin, Matrigel: basement membrane matrix with biological activity. *Seminars in Cancer Biology*, 2005. 15(5): p. 378-386.
[106] Griffith, L.G. and M.A. Swartz, Capturing complex 3D tissue physiology in vitro. *Nature Reviews Molecular Cell Biology*, 2006. 7(3): p. 211-224.
[107] Langer, R. and D.A. Tirrell, Designing materials for biology and medicine. *Nature*, 2004. 428(6982): p. 487-492.
[108] Elisseeff, J., et al., Transdermal photopolymerization for minimally invasive implantation. *Proceedings of the National Academy of Sciences*, 1999. 96(6): p. 3104-3107.

[109] Moon, S., et al., Layer by layer three-dimensional tissue epitaxy by cell-laden hydrogel droplets. *Tissue Engineering Part C: Methods,* 2010. 16(1): p. 157-166.

[110] Xu, F., et al., A three-dimensional in vitro ovarian cancer coculture model using a high-throughput cell patterning platform. *Biotechnology Journal,* 2011. 6(2): p. 204-212.

[111] Chaabane, S., et al., Periosteal chondrosarcoma. *American Journal of Roentgenology,* 2009. 192(1): p. W1-6.

[112] Tiet, T., et al., Constitutive hedgehog signaling in chondrosarcoma up-regulates tumor cell proliferation. *The American Journal of Pathology,* 2006. 168(1): p. 321 - 30.

[113] Parsch, D., et al., Consequences of telomerase inhibition by BIBR1532 on proliferation and chemosensitivity of chondrosarcoma cell lines. *Cancer Investigation,* 2008. 26(6): p. 590-596.

[114] Kim, D., et al., siRNA-based targeting of antiapoptotic genes can reverse chemoresistance in P-glycoprotein expressing chondrosarcoma cells. *Mol. Cancer,* 2009. 8: p. 28.

[115] Miyaji, T., et al., Monoclonal antibody to parathyroid hormone-related protein induces differentiation and apoptosis of chondrosarcoma cells. *Cancer Letters,* 2003. 199(2): p. 147-155.

[116] Kim, D.W., et al., Targeting of cell survival genes using small interfering RNAs (siRNAs) enhances radiosensitivity of grade II chondrosarcoma cells. *Journal of Orthopaedic Research,* 2007. 25(6): p. 820-828.

[117] Anne Gomez-Brouchet, Frédéric Mourcin, Pierre-Antoine Gourraud et al., Galectin-1 is a powerful marker to distinguish chondroblastic osteosarcoma and conventional chondrosarcoma. *Human Pathology,* 41(9): p. 1220-1230.

[118] Matsuura, S., Oda Y., Matono H. et al., Overexpression of A disintegrin and metalloproteinase 28 is correlated with high histologic grade in conventional chondrosarcoma. 2011, 41(3): p. 343-351.

In: Sarcoma
Editor: Eric J. Butler

ISBN: 978-1-62100-362-5
© 2012 Nova Science Publishers, Inc.

Chapter V

The Potential of Suicide Plus Immune Gene Therapy for Treating Osteosarcoma: The Experience on Canine Veterinary Patients

Liliana M. E. Finocchiaro, Agustina Spector, Ursula A. Rossi, María L. Gil-Cardeza, José L. Suarez, María D. Riveros, Marcela S. Villaverde and Gerardo C. Glikin
Instituto de Oncología "Ángel H. Roffo", Universidad de Buenos Aires, Buenos Aires, Argentina

Abstract

Comparative oncology amalgamates the experience on naturally occurring cancers in veterinary patients into more general studies of cancer, especially those focused on the human disease. Naturally occurring tumors in dogs have clinical and biological similarities to human cancers that are difficult to replicate in other model systems.

Osteosarcoma (OSA) accounts for approximately 85% of primary bone cancers in the dog. It is a common cancer of large to giant breed dogs, and it occurs primarily in the appendicular skeleton. Being a common and highly metastatic tumor, it does not have additional treatment options when adjuvant chemotherapy has failed against its disseminated form. Even with removal of the primary tumor, before spread of the cancer is clinically detectable, metastases to lung, bone, or other sites eventually develop in almost all dogs. Palliative radiation therapy for bone pain is indicated in those dogs that do not undergo amputation or a limb-sparing surgery. Standard treatments result in median survival rates ranging between 78 and 130 days.

In such context the need to develop new treatments to fight OSA is compelling. While most of cancer gene therapy for canine veterinary patients was aimed to spontaneous melanoma and some to primary canine soft-tissue sarcomas, only one was specifically aimed to OSA. Therefore, we propose a new treatment combining: (i) the local antiproliferative effects of interferon-β and HSV-thymidine kinase suicide gene therapy with (ii) the systemic effects triggered by OSA antigens in an immunostimulatory environment created by the slow secretion of granulocyte and macrophage colony-stimulating factor and interleukin-2.

Beyond the high safety standard of the proposed treatment on six canine osteosarcoma patients, four of them survived more than 6 months (among them, two exceeded 1 year). In addition, the treatment prevented or delayed local relapse, regional metastases and distant metastases, suggesting a strong systemic antitumor immunity.

We are presenting detailed evidences of two cases of a very successful outcome: (i) a first one presenting a long term recurrence-free period after tumor surgical excision and (ii) a second one of a long-lasting complete remission without surgical intervention.

As a conclusion of this work we suggest that the use of this treatment, associated or not to the surgical removal of the tumor (depending on the initial stage of the disease), would be safe and could delay or prevent recurrence and metastases, with the consequent quality of life and survival rate improvement. To establish the treatment efficacy, the encouraging results presented here warrant the proposal of a subsequent trial including a representative amount of canine patients.

Introduction

Osteosarcoma in dogs and humans is strikingly similar in its clinical presentation, biology, treatment, complications, and outcomes (although human patients do better). Translational research and treatment are therefore particularly fruitful for this disease, despite some differences between the species (Withrow and Wilkins, 2010).

Human osteosarcoma, which is the most common malignant primary bone tumor, occurs most frequently in adolescents, but there is a second incidence peak among individuals aged >60 years. Thirty percent of patients with localized disease and eighty percent of patients with metastatic disease at diagnosis will relapse. Most osteosarcoma epidemiology studies have been embedded in large analyses of all bone tumors or focused on cases occurring in adolescence. While survival rates vary by anatomic site and disease stage, despite the availability of new treatments like multiagent chemotherapy combined with aggressive surgical resection, they did not improve significantly from 1984 to 2004 (Mirabello et al., 2009). Even though lymph node metastasis is rare, human osteosarcoma most often metastasizes to the lung and bone. At diagnosis, approximately 80% of patients are believed to have micrometastatic disease, but only 8-15% are properly diagnosed. The 5-year survival rate is between 65% and 75% for localized disease, whereas for patients with metastasis at presentation, it remains poor at 20% (Mueller *et al.* 2007)

On the other hand, osteosarcoma (OSA) accounts for approximately 85% of primary bone cancers in the dog (Mayer and Grier, 2006). It is a common cancer of large to giant breed dogs, and it occurs primarily in the appendicular skeleton. OSA in dogs is a common and highly metastatic tumor that does not have additional treatment options when adjuvant chemotherapy has failed against its disseminated form (Dow et al., 2005). Even with removal of the primary tumor before spread of the cancer is clinically detectable, metastases to lung, bone, or other sites eventually develop in almost all dogs (Mayer and Grier, 2006). Histologically confirmed regional lymph node metastases were found only in about 4% of dogs with osteosarcoma at the time of limb amputation. Although less than 15% of dogs have radiographically detectable pulmonary metastases at initial evaluation, occult metastatic disease is present in approximately 90% of dogs at presentation (Mueller et al., 2007). Palliative radiation therapy for bone pain is indicated in those dogs that do not undergo amputation or a limb-sparing surgery.

The parallels between canine and human osteosarcoma are perhaps the strongest across the comparative oncology opportunities (Gorlick and Khanna, 2010). Both diseases are characterized by primary tumor growth in the appendicular skeleton and a high risk for metastasis to the lungs. The canine disease is indistinguishable from the human disease at the histologic and gene expression levels. Indeed, both conventional and investigational treatments for both the primary tumor and the metastatic disease are associated with similar response features in both species. The primary differences between the models are the age of development and the prevalence of disease. In dogs, osteosarcoma is a disease of older, large breed dogs (i.e., 6 to 12 years of age), whereas osteosarcoma occurs most commonly in the second decade of life in humans. The high prevalence and the relatively rapid rate of disease progression (median disease-free interval following surgery alone is 4 months; with surgery and chemotherapy, 13 months) provides the opportunity to evaluate novel treatment options in dogs in a relatively compressed time period.

Gene therapy for human osteosarcoma is gaining additional momentum with the introduction of delivery vehicles such as hydrogels and modified adenoviral vectors (Broadhead et al., 2010). With safer gene-delivery vehicles being produced, nucleic acid-based therapeutic constructs are becoming more amenable to clinical application. Targets such as ezrin, uPAR and PEDF have been shown to be efficacious for osteosarcoma in animal models. A combination of gene therapy and conventional therapies may yet achieve more complete disease control and warrants further evaluation for osteosarcoma.

Until nowadays, few attempts were made to use a gene therapy approach to fight canine osteosarcoma (Finocchiaro and Glikin, 2008[a]). Beyond the early attempts with irradiated hGM-CSF producing autologous tumor cells plasmid transferred by gene gun (Hogge et al., 1998), only two additional articles reported additional data. OSA lung metastases were safely treated by systemic gene delivery via intravenous injection of cationic liposome-DNA complexes carrying canine IL-2 gene (Dow et al., 2005). On the other hand, OSA primary or locally recurrent tumors were treated by combining suicide gene plus immunogene therapy, in the same way as it currently is presented in this chapter (Finocchiaro et al., 2011).

It was already shown that, in dogs with melanoma, intratumor injections of lipid-complexed plasmid DNA encoding the herpes simplex virus thymidine kinase (HSVtk) suicide gene sensitized transfected cells to ganciclovir (GCV) (Finocchiaro et al., 2008). The administration of irradiated xenogeneic cells genetically modified to secrete human interleukin-2 (hIL-2) and human granulocyte-macrophage colony-stimulating factor (hGM-CSF), together with formolized tumor extracts to dogs with melanoma was proposed as a co-adjuvant of suicide gene therapy and a booster of the immune response against melanoma (Finocchiaro and Glikin, 2008[b]). This strategy halted the state of relative immune tolerance and promoted a strong immune response against a broader array of tumor antigens, leading to an inhibition of tumor growth, or tumor rejection. The repeated induction of a potent localized immune stimulus by xenoantigens, together with the secretion of cytokines by γ-irradiated engineered xenogeneic cells, was able to elicit a powerful antitumor response. It is noteworthy that immunotherapy, in combination with suicide gene therapy, holds the most promise for malignant melanoma patients with minimal residual disease after surgery (Finocchiaro and Glikin, 2008[b]). This surgery adjuvant treatment controlled tumor growth, delaying or preventing post-surgical recurrence and distant metastasis, significantly extended survival and recovered the quality of life.

Local expression of interferon-β (IFN-β) inhibits angiogenesis (Streck et al., 2006) and tumor growth by direct cytotoxicity (Yoshida et al., 2004), as well as it increases tumor cell immunogenicity and antitumor immune response. Human sarcoma cell lines were reported as sensitive to the HSV*tk*/GCV system (Veldwijk et al., 2004) and preliminary *in vitro* data obtained in our laboratory showed that canine melanoma (Gil-Cardeza et al. 2010) or sarcoma spheroids that were resistant to the HSV*tk*/GCV system resulted highly sensitive to canine IFN-β (cIFN-β) gene transfer. Thus, before starting a controlled trial on the effects of the combination of local suicide gene therapy plus cIFN-β with a systemic anti-cancer vaccine in canine spontaneous osteosarcoma patients, we evaluated the feasibility and safety of this combination as main treatment or as adjuvant of surgery.

Materials and Methods

Plasmids

Plasmids psCMV*tk* (4.5 Kb) and psCMVcIFNβ (3.9 Kb) carry respectively HSV*tk* (1.2 Kb) and cIFN-β (0.6 Kb) in the polylinker site of psCMV (3.3 Kb), downstream of the CMV promoter and upstream of poly A sequences, and the kanamycin resistance gene for selection in *E. coli*. Plasmids were grown, chromatographically purified and quality assessed as described (Finocchiaro and Glikin, 2008[b]). Plasmid DNA for injection was resuspended to a final concentration of 2.0 mg ml^{-1} in sterile PBS.

Liposome Preparation and in Vivo Lipofection

Liposomes for injection were prepared by combining equimolar amounts of DMRIE (kindly provided by BioSidus SA, Buenos Aires, Argentina) and DOPE (Sigma, St Louis, MO, USA) and treated as described (Finocchiaro and Glikin, 2008[b]). Before injection, liposomes and equal amounts of plasmid DNAs (1:2 v:v) were mixed and allowed to combine at room temperature for 10 min. Then GCV (Richet SA, Buenos Aires, Argentina; 5 mg mg^{-1} DNA) was added. The mixture was injected intra- and/or peritumorally at multiple sites at a final volume of 1-4 ml, depending on tumor size.

Tumor Vaccines Preparation

Autologous and/or allogeneic tumor cell preparations were prepared for subcutaneous injection as described (Finocchiaro et al. 2011).

Patients

Dogs entered into the study had confirmed histopathological diagnosis of osteosarcoma. All dogs were determined to be free of other severe underlying systemic illnesses. During the study, dogs did not receive chemotherapy or another potentially antitumor or immunosuppressive medication. When needed, standard antibiotics, non steroid anti-inflammatory and/or analgesic medication was administered. The dogs' owners were notified about the experimental nature of the treatment, and all of them granted written informed consent for treatment. Specially trained veterinary professionals, working in accordance with the laws and regulations of our country (Argentina), performed the treatment. All scientific and ethical issues related to the veterinary clinical trial were evaluated and approved by the appropriate committee of the granting agency (ANPCYT, Argentina).

Treatment

Four of 6 patients were subjected to complete or cytoreductive surgery. When possible, the surgical margin of the cavity after tumor removal was infiltrated with HSV*tk* and cIFN-β carrying lipoplexes co-delivered with GCV evenly distributed at multiple sites in the surrounding areas and/or in the residual tumor mass. Between 5 and 10 days after surgery, patients were clinically controlled and treated once a week for 5 weeks with a subcutaneous vaccine containing autologous or allogeneic formolized tumor fragments (containing about 50-100 µl of insoluble pellet). Patients without local disease continued the treatment only with *s.c.* vaccine: 5 times (5X) weekly, 5X biweekly, 5X monthly and finally every 3 months until relapse or death. Patients with local disease (unresectable or partially removed tumor, unsafe surgery limits or with postsurgical relapse received in the remaining tumor or adjacent areas multiple injections of lipoplexes carrying equal amounts of psCMV*tk* plus psCMV-IFNβ (1-4 mg DNA) co-delivered with GCV (5-20 mg) according to tumor size (about 0.1 mg DNA.cm^{-2} of surgical margin). They continued with the chronic treatment or until disappearance of any evidence of local disease. At this point, they followed the previous scheme. The follow-up lasted until the patients' death. Periodic clinical evaluations were performed on every day of treatment and were completed by monthly or bimonthly clinical laboratory analysis. Thoracic radiographs and abdominal echographs were done before treatment and every month according to the patients' response and at longer intervals in long-term surviving animals. Evaluation of the effects on the quality of life was based on the owner's response to a questionnaire completed during every treatment session. Two patients were subjected to the combined treatment without previous surgery.

Tumor Response Criteria

Tumor responses were classified as complete remission (CR), macroscopic disappearance of the tumor; partial remission (PR), reduction of tumor size by more than 50%; stable disease (SD), stabilization or increase in tumor size up to 50% for at least 125 days after start of treatment; progressive disease, increase of tumor size higher than 50%. Assessment of clinical response has taken into account all measurable lesions. Only CR and PR were considered to determine the objective response rate. CR, PR and SD were included to determine tumor control rate. Tumor volumes (evaluated by caliper measuring three diameters) were calculated as $4/3\pi r_1 r_2 r_3$.

Results

Patients' Demographics

As depicted in Table 1, most of the canine osteosarcoma patients (3 males, 3 females) were aged (5 out of 6) with an average age of about 13 years (patient 1 excluded). Three breeds were represented among patients: German Shepherd (2), Dogue de Bordeaux (1) and Rottweiler (2). Three tumors were located at the limbs and 3 at the head.

Table1. Patients demographics

Patient #	Breed	Age (Years)	Sex	Weight(Kg)	Site
1	Dogue de Bordeaux	3	male	64	forearm
2	Rottweiler	9	female	45	forearm
3	German Shepherd	10	female	35	forefoot
4	German Shepherd	12	male	32	head
5	Mixed	15	female	20	head
6	Pekingese	18	male	6	head

Patients' Treatment Outcome

Combination of suicide gene therapy with immunotherapy has shown to provide consistent benefit for local and systemic control of canine tumors (Finocchiaro et al., 2008; Finocchiaro and Glikin, 2008[b]; Finocchiaro et al., 2011). It is noteworthy that the suicide gene-generated margin played a critical role abolishing local relapse in 49%, or delaying it (from 56 to 148 days) in 19% of the treated melanoma patients (Finocchiaro and Glikin, 2008[b]). The beneficial role of additional local treatment with IFN-β has not been evaluated at that time, but encouraging results were obtained treating different canine sarcomas (Finocchiaro et al., 2011). The present study evaluated the feasibility and safety of a new combined treatment for spontaneous canine osteosarcoma.

Patient 1: A 3 year-old Dogue de Bordeaux male weighting 64 Kg was evaluated because of progressive left arm pain and lameness increasing progressively during 8 weeks. Radiographic analysis of the left shoulder revealed a proliferative lesion and loss of normal trabecular architecture within the proximal metaphysis at the left humerus head (Figure 1, upper left panel).

Table 2. Patients treatment outcome

Patient #	1st Local Treat.	Local Relapse	2nd Local Treat.	VAX	Response Local Tumor	Lymph Node	Mts	SURVIVAL (Days)	Cause of Death
1	PT	No	-	ALV	CR	-	-	>453	Alive
2	CX+PT	No	-	AUV	-	-	+	609	Related to OSA
3	IT	-	-	ALV	PR	-	-	96	Unrelated to OSA
4	CX	Yes	CX+PT	AUV	-	SD	-	193	Related to OSA
5	CX+PT	No	-	AUV	-	-	-	226	Unrelated to OSA
6	CX	Yes	IT	ALV	-	SD	-	157	Related to OSA

CX: surgery; IT: intratumor cIFN-β + suicide genes injection; PT: peritumoral cIFN-β + suicide genes injection / VAX: vaccine; ALV: allogeneic; AUV: autologous / CR: complete response; PR: partial response; SD: stable disease; MTS: distant metastasis / OSA: osteosarcoma. Data about patients 3 to 6 as published (Finocchiaro et al., 2011).

Lateral thoracic radiographs showed no evidence of lung metastasis. The biopsy of the lesion was diagnosed as osteoblastic osteosarcoma by histopathological analysis. A biochemical analysis and urinalysis were performed at that time, and results were unremarkable. The owner declined palliative amputation of the left arm. In this case no chemotherapy was performed, and local treatment only comprised local peritumoral injections of ganciclovir and lipoplexes carrying suicide plus cIFNβ genes. Simultaneously an allogeneic vaccine preparation was applied for systemic control of the disease. Most of the signs of pain disappeared 4 weeks after starting treatment, with a progressive recovery of patient's shoulder function. Survey radiography was performed 3 months after starting treatment (Figure 1, upper right panel) and revealed considerable resolution of the previous lesion. There was no swelling or signs of pain in the area of the prior mass. Periodic radiological images paralleled this clinical outcome showing a steady regression of the lesion that was fairly noted after 4 months of treatment. Nine months after the beginning of treatment, radiography of the left shoulder revealed the restoration of normal cortex surface on the humerus head with almost complete resolution of the previous lesion displaying only a smooth sclerotic periosteal reaction at the site (Figure 1, lower right panel). No clinical or radiological evidence of local or systemic disease was detected on the 10th month of treatment (Figure 1, lower left panel). The owner reported that the dog was free of clinical signs of disease and fully recovered his quality of life.

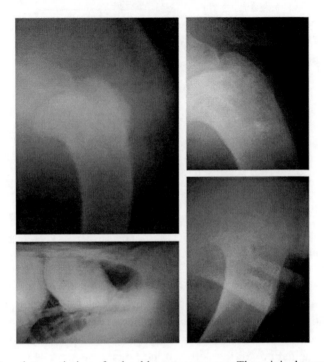

Figure 1. Complete remission of a shoulder osteosarcoma: The original tumor at the time of diagnosis (upper left panel) displayed a noticeable remission 3 months after starting the combined gene therapy treatment (upper right panel) and almost completely disappeared after 9 months of treatment (lower right panel). Lateral thoracic radiograph showed no evidence of metastatic disease on the 10th month (lower left panel).

Patient 2: A 9 year-old Rottweiler female weighting 45 Kg was evaluated because of progressive right forelimb lameness during 6 weeks. On physical examination, a firm swelling in the distal portion of the ulna, right arm pain and claudication were evident. A biochemical analysis and urinalysis were performed at that time, and results were within normal range, with the exception of a mild increase in alkaline phosphatase activity. Radiography of the right radius and ulna was performed and revealed a combined destructive and proliferative lesion and loss of normal trabecular architecture within at the medial/distal diaphysis of the ulna (Figure 2 upper left panel). Initial thoracic radiography did not reveal evidence of pulmonary metastatic disease. The biopsy of the lesion was diagnosed by histopathological analysis as high-grade angioblastic osteosarcoma. Then, limb sparing surgery was indicated. The patient was subjected to partial ulna osteotomy (tumor mean diameter 4.5 cm, mean height 6.0 cm) with surgical margins of about 2 cm and resection of compromised soft issues (Figure 2 upper right panel). The radius surface facing the ulna was scraped off, without establishing safe surgical margins on the remaining bone. Surgical margins were injected with lipoplexes carrying suicide plus cIFNβ genes. Only one post-surgical session of *i.v.* carboplatin (300 mg/m^2) chemotherapy was performed before autologous tumor vaccination.

As followed by periodical forelimb and chest radiography, no local relapse or lung metastatic disease was observed for more than 18 months) after starting the treatment (Figure 2 lower right panel). The owner reported that the dog was free of clinical signs of disease. Nevertheless, about 17 months after surgery, pain followed by paraplegia linked to osteolysis at the level of L2 as evidenced by radiography (Figure 2 lower left panel). Being the metastatic disease the probable cause of these symptoms together with the age of the patient, the owner did not allow further local treatment.

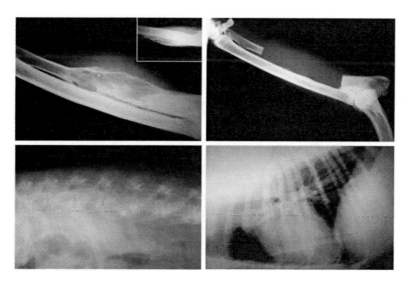

Figure 2. Absence of local relapse of a forelimb osteosarcoma: The original tumor at the time of diagnosis (lateral view: upper left panel, frontal view: inset) did not display recurrence up to 18 months days after starting the combined gene therapy treatment (upper right panel). Lateral thoracic radiograph showed no evidence of metastatic disease at the same date (lower right panel). Bone metastasis at the level of L2 was diagnosed 17 months after starting treatment (lower left panel).

Patient 3: A 10 year-old German Shepherd female weighting 35 Kg was subjected to palliative amputation of the right forelimb because of osteosarcoma. No gene therapy treatment was performed in that occasion. Later on, a second tumor appeared on the left radius. Intratumor injections of lipoplexes containing cIFN-β/suicide genes, together with *s.c.* allogeneic vaccine produced a partial response with restoration of normal bone density at the tumor region as evidenced by radiographic images. During treatment, local swelling and pain diminished improving the patient's quality of life. Unfortunately over time the combination of the amputation and overweight diminished the rear feet functionality with the subsequent loss of activity and quality of life. Finally, the patient was humanely euthanized by decision of its owners 3 months after starting the treatment.

Patient 4: A 12 year-old German Shepherd male weighting 32 Kg was subjected to surgical removal of an osteosarcoma (tumor mean diameter 5.7 cm, mean height 2.6 cm) on the left maxilla. Because of the location, no safe surgical margins could be established and it was not possible to inject the bone next to the tumor. Then, lipoplexes containing cIFN-β/suicide genes were injected in the soft tissue surrounding the tumor area. During the cycle of five weekly *s.c.* autologous vaccine, the tumor reappeared and an additional surgery was performed. This poorly responsive pattern occurred again and a third surgery was performed. After 6 months of periodical vaccination, the ipsilateral lymph node was reactive (about 2.0 cm diameter) without evidence of metastatic spread of the disease to lungs as detected by radiographic images. Due to the lack of a local disease free interval between surgical procedures and despite the good quality of life observed between surgeries, the owners decided humanely euthanize the patient.

Patient 5: A 15 year-old Mixed breed female weighting 20 Kg was subjected to surgical removal of an osteosarcoma (tumor mean diameter: 1.8 cm) in the mandible. The suicide gene-generated margin and the *s.c.* autologous vaccine precluded post-surgical recurrence for more than 7 months, when the patient died due to an unrelated disease.

Patient 6: A 18 year-old Pekingese male weighting 6 Kg was subjected to surgical removal of an osteosarcoma (tumor mean diameter: 2.4 cm) in the palate. The suicide gene-generated margin and the *s.c.* autologous vaccine succeeded in preventing post-surgical relapse for more than 5 months. Then, the ipsilateral lymph node was reactive (about 3.0 cm diameter) without evidence of metastatic spread of the disease to lungs detected by radiographic images. The owners refused any additional treatment and decided humanely euthanize the patient.

Discussion

Multiple injections into the tumor beds (or surrounding areas) of the lipoplexes carrying cIFN-β and suicide gene plus gancyclovir, together with the subcutaneous administration of cytokine-secreting autologous or allogeneic vaccine, resulted feasible, safe and non-allergenic and could be applied repeatedly. Undesirable side effects such as systemic toxicity, organ dysfunction or fever were not found in any patient. Significant changes in complete blood counts or serum biochemical parameters were not observed.

Four osteosarcoma cases were subjected to surgery as first local treatment. Even though surgery excision was often incomplete because of the tumor location, the proposed treatment prevented or delayed local recurrence in three patients. This decrease in the recurrence rate was probably due to four factors. First, the surgical margin of the cavity left after removing the tumor was infiltrated with a lipid-complexed plasmid bearing cIFN-β and suicide genes co-administered with ganciclovir (ISG), evenly distributed at multiple sites in the margin. This ISG generated new margin significantly delayed or prevented postsurgical recurrence of the tumors (Finocchiaro and Glikin, 2008[b]). Secondly, injections of lipid-complexed ISG into the tumor area would circumvent tolerance and immunosuppression mediated by the tumor, providing an immunostimulatory microenvironment necessary for immune cells activated by the vaccine to destroy more efficiently the residual tumor. Immunostimulatory sequences in the plasmid DNA, the cationic lipids and cIFN-β expression would have increased the immunogenicity of the tumor. Thirdly, as a co-adjuvant to the ISG therapy and to boost the immune response against the osteosarcoma, a subcutaneous autologous or allogeneic vaccine enhanced by the local slow release of hGM-CSF and hIL-2 was administered as it was proposed for melanoma (Finocchiaro and Glikin, 2008[b]). This whole-tumor vaccine would have immunized the canine patients against a broad array of tumor surface antigens, increasing the likelihood of effective immunostimulation. The potential of immunotherapy for osteosarcamoma was suggested by the fact that, in dogs with osteosarcoma treated with limb-salvage surgery, infection has a positive influence on survival (Lascelles *et al.*, 2005). In addition, the lack of lung metastatic spread of the disease in all our treated patients supports the strong involvement of all local and systemic immune stimulating effects.

Finally, the combined treatment did not produce significant adverse side effects. The injection of IFN-β lipoplexes, that were described as safe in a pilot study for human melanoma (Matsumoto et al., 2008), showed a safety profile similar to the combined gene therapy treatment for canine melanoma reported previously (Finocchiaro and Glikin, 2008[b]).

In the case of advanced canine OSA, it was reported that a combination of surgery and chemotherapy allowed a median survival time of 78 days, and palliative radiation and chemotherapy produced a statistically significant a longer median survival time of 130 days (Boston et al. 2004). Following our approach, 2 primary OSA treated locally displayed objective responses (PT: complete, IT: partial) and 2 lymph node metastases displayed temporary stable disease. OSA was transiently controlled in all the patients (1 surviving more than 1.5 year, 2 more than 6 months and 1 more than 5 months) while they maintained a good quality of life. In addition, no evidence of disease after treatment was observed in the case of complete remission for more than 1.2 year.

In conclusion, the use of this treatment after surgical removal of the tumor is safe and could delay or prevent post-surgical recurrence and metastases, with the consequent quality of life and survival rate improvement. In addition, when diagnosed at the early stages, a peritumoral application of interferon-β plus suicide genes in combination with subcutaneous vaccine could be effective in controlling both local (recurrence) and distant disease (metastases).

Our combined approach holds great promise as a novel gene therapy strategy to treat both canine and human osteosarcoma. A subsequent trial including a representative amount of osteosarcoma canine patients is being currently tested to establish the efficacy of the treatment.

Acknowledgments

We are grateful to our patients and their owners for their cooperation and participation in this study. We thank G. Zenobi for technical assistance, VMD M. Maminska and VMD F. Calcagno for patients' treatment and care, and VMD D. de Simone for expert reading of radiographies.

This work was partially supported by grants from ANPCYT/FONCYT PICT 2007-00539, CONICET PIP 2008 and UBACYT PID 2008-M027. L.M.E.F. and G.C.G. are investigators, and M.L.G-C. and M.S.V., are fellows of the Consejo Nacional de Investigaciones Científicas y Técnicas (CONICET, Argentina). A.S. and J.L.S. are VMDs working in veterinary private practice.

References

Broadhead ML, Clark JC, Choong PF, Dass CR. Making gene therapy for osteosarcoma a reality. *Expert Rev. Anticancer Ther.* 2010; *10:* 477-480.

Dow S, Elmslie R, Kurzman I, MacEwen G, Pericle F, Liggitt D. Phase I study of liposome-DNA complexes encoding the interleukin-2 gene in dogs with osteosarcoma lung metastases. *Hum. Gene. Ther.* 2005; *16:* 937-946.

Finocchiaro LME, Glikin, GC. Cancer gene therapy in large animals. In New Gene Therapy and Cancer Research, W.B. Gustafsson (Ed.). Nova Science Publishers, Inc. (New York, U.S.A.). pp. 279-292 (2008). ISBN: 1-60021-969-1. [a].

Finocchiaro LME, Glikin GC. Cytokine-enhanced vaccine and suicide gene therapy as surgery adjuvant treatments for spontaneous canine melanoma. *Gene. Ther.* 2008; *15:* 267-276. [b]

Finocchiaro LME., Fiszman GL, Karara AL, Glikin GC. Suicide gene and cytokines combined non viral gene therapy for canine spontaneous melanoma. *Cancer Gene. Ther.* 2008; *15:* 165-172.

Finocchiaro LME, Villaverde MS, Gil-Cardeza ML, Riveros MD, Glikin GC: Cytokine-enhanced vaccine and interferon-β plus suicide gene as combined therapy for spontaneous canine sarcomas. *Res. Vet. Sci.* 2011 *91:* 230-234.

Gil-Cardeza ML, Villaverde MS, Fiszman GL, Altamirano NA, Cwirenbaum RA, Glikin GC, Finocchiaro LME. Suicide gene therapy on spontaneous canine melanoma: correlations between *in vivo* tumors and their derived multicell spheroids *in vitro*. *Gene. Ther.* 2010; *17:* 26-36.

Gorlick R, Khanna C. Osteosarcoma. *J. Bone Miner. Res.* 2010; *25:* 683-691.

Hogge GS, Burkholder JK, Culp J, Albertini MR, Dubielzig RR, Keller ET, Yang NS, MacEwen EG. Development of human granulocyte-macrophage colony-stimulating factor-transfected tumor cell vaccines for the treatment of spontaneous canine cancer. *Human Gene Ther.* 1998; *9:* 1851-1861.

Lascelles BD, Dernell WS, Correa MT, Lafferty M, Devitt CM, Kuntz CA, Straw RC, Withrow SJ. Improved survival associated with postoperative wound infection in dogs treated with limb-salvage surgery for osteosarcoma. *Ann. Surg. Oncol.* 2005; *12:* 1073-1083.

Matsumoto K, Kubo H, Murata H, Uhara H, Takata M, Shibata S, Yasue S, Sakakibara A, Tomita Y, Kageshita T, Kawakami Y, Mizuno M. Yoshida J, Saida T. A pilot study of human interferon beta gene therapy for patients with advanced melanoma by *in vivo* transduction using cationic liposomes, *Jpn. J. Clin. Oncol.* 2008; *38:* 849-856.

Mayer, M.N., Grier, C.K., Palliative radiation therapy for canine osteosarcoma. *Can. Vet. J.* 2006; *47:* 707-709.

Mirabello L, Troisi RJ, Savage SA. Osteosarcoma incidence and survival rates from 1973 to 2004: data from the Surveillance, Epidemiology, and End Results Program. *Cancer.* 2009; *115:* 1531-1543.

Mueller F, Fuchs B, Kaser-Hotz B. Comparative biology of human and canine osteosarcoma. *Anticancer Res.* 2007; *27:* 155-164.

Streck CJ, Dickson PV, Ng CY, Zhou J, Hall MM, Gray JT, Nathwani AC, Davidoff AM, Antitumor efficacy of AAV-mediated systemic delivery of interferon-beta. *Cancer Gene Ther.* 2006; *13:* 99-106.

Veldwijk MR, Berlinghoff S, Laufs S, Hengge UR, Zeller WJ, Wenz F, Fruehauf S. Suicide gene therapy of sarcoma cell lines using recombinant adeno-associated virus 2 vectors. *Cancer Gene Ther.* 2004; *11:* 577-584.

Withrow SJ, Wilkins RM. Cross talk from pets to people: translational osteosarcoma treatments *ILAR J.* 2010; *51:* 208-213.

Yoshida J, Mizuno M, Wakabayashi T. Interferon-beta gene therapy for cancer: basic research to clinical application. *Cancer Sci.* 2004; *95:* 858-865.

In: Sarcoma
Editor: Eric J. Butler

ISBN: 978-1-62100-362-5
© 2012 Nova Science Publishers, Inc.

Chapter VI

New Concept of Limb Salvage Surgery in Musculoskeletal Sarcomas with Acridine Orange Therapy

Katsuyuki Kusuzaki[1,2,7], Shigekuni Hosogi[2], Eishi Ashihara[2], Takao Matsubara[3], Haruhiko Satonaka[3], Tomoki Nakamura[3], Akihiko Matsumine[3], Akihiro Sudo[3], Atsumasa Uchida[3], Hiroaki Murata[4], Nicola Baldini[5], Stefano Fais[6] and Yoshinori Marunaka[2,7]

[1]Department of Orthopedic Surgery, Kyoto Kujo Hospital, Kyoto, Japan
[2]Department of Molecular Cell Physiology, Kyoto Prefectural University of Medicine, Graduate School of Medical Science, Kyoto, Japan
[3]Department of Orthopedic Surgery, Mie University Graduate School of Medicine, Tsu, Mie, Japan
[4]Department of Orthopedic Surgery, Matsushita Memorial Hospital, Osaka Japan
[5]Laboratory of Orthopaedic Pathophysiology and Regenerative Medicine, Università di Bologna-Alma Mater Studiorum and Istituto Ortopedico Rizzoli, Bologna, Italy
[6]Department of Therapeutic Research and Medicines Evaluation of Istituto Superiore di Sanità, Rome, Italy
[7]Japan Institute for Food Education and Health, Heian Jogakuin (St. Agnes') University, Kyoto, Japan

Abstract

Although limb salvage surgery involving wide resection and limb reconstruction for musculoskeletal sarcomas is well established for low risk of local tumor recurrence, limb function is unsatisfactory for many patients because of the disability in active athletics such as running, jumping, throwing, swimming etc. To avoid poor limb function caused by surgery, it is important to preserve normal nerves, vessels, bones, joints and muscles adjacent to tumor as possible as we can, supported by effective adjuvant therapy to inhibit local tumor recurrence.

To develop minimally-invasive limb salvage surgery with minimal damage of normal tissues and low risk of local recurrence, we have recently established a new limb salvage modality of acridine orange (AO) therapy (AOT) based on photodynamic surgery (PDS), photodynamic therapy (PDT) and radiodynamic therapy (RDT) using AO in patients with high-grade malignant musculoskeletal sarcoma. Clinical outcomes of the study showed that: 1) low risk of local recurrence which is almost the same as that with conventional wide resection, and 2) superior limb function to that by wide resection.

In this chapter, we present mechanisms of cytocidal effects of AOT based on experimental research and clinical outcome of AOT applied to musculoskeletal sarcoma patients.

Introduction

Limb salvage surgery with wide tumor resection followed by limb reconstruction using various types of endoprosthesis or biological materials such as bone allo/autograft, free vascularized fibula, in situ autograft treated with heat or nitrogen liquid, autograft of vessels, nerves, tendons and muscles, etc for the treatment of musculoskeletal sarcomas has advanced remarkably over the last 40 years [1, 2]. However, recovery of limb function has not yet been satisfactorily achieved, and most of the treated patients are still not capable of running and swimming fast, jumping well, or throwing a ball far in sports activity. Since these disabilities markedly interfere with the quality of life of the patients, especially in children or young people, methods for achieving satisfactory recovery of limb function after limb salvage surgery need to be explored urgently [3, 4, 5, 6].

For this purpose, we have been studying the development and establishment of acridine orange therapy (AOT) which consists of three procedures of photodynamic surgery (PDS), photodynamic therapy (PDT) and radiodynamic therapy (RDT) with AO after tumor excision with minimal damage of normal tissues, for musculoskeletal sarcoma since 1990.

AO was extracted as a weak basic dye from coal tar over a hundred years ago. It has various unique biological activities and has been shown to be a useful fluorescent dye specific for DNA and RNA [7, 8], a pH indicator [9], photosensitizer [10, 11], antitumor [12, 13] and anti-malarial drug [14], and detector of bacteria and parasites [14, 15]. Our studies revealed that AO selectively accumulates into musculoskeletal sarcomas and that after illumination of the tumors with visible light or irradiation with low-dose X-rays, the dye rapidly exerts selective cytocidal effects against the sarcoma cells [16-27]. Therefore, we have been applying minimal invasive surgery combined with AOT to human musculoskeletal sarcomas, in order to preserve an excellent limb function with low risk of local tumor recurrence as well as good prognosis.

In this review, we present results of in vitro and in vivo basic research of AO-PDT and AO-RDT using mouse osteosarcoma model and outcome of the clinical application of AOT to musculoskeletal sarcoma patients [23-28].

Basic Research

1. Selective Accumulation of AO in Mouse Osteosarcoma Cells

Results of our basic studies using mouse osteosarcoma cells have revealed that AO binds densely as dimer form to lysosomes and other acidic vesicles including endosomes, phagosomes, secretion granules, etc., emitting orange fluorescence after blue light excitation in living cultured mouse osteosarcoma cells and sparsely binds as monomer form to RNAs in cytoplasm (transfer RNA and micro RNA or ribosomal RNA) and nucleolus (messenger RNA), emitting green fluorescence. AO does not accumulate into other organelles of mitochondria, Golgi apparatus or endoplasmic reticulum [17, 20, 29].

In an in vivo study using mouse osteosarcoma model, in which culture cells were subcutaneously transplanted at the back skin, the tumor emitted strong green fluorescence at 2 hours after intraperitoneal (10mg/kg) or intravenous injection (1mg/kg) of AO followed by blue excitation, while normal muscle and adipose tissue cells did not. Therefore, the tumor could be clearly visualized by fluorescence under the fluorescence surgical microscope equipped with high resolution CCD camera (fluorovisualization effect) [17, 18, 21]. Even in a small lesion of multiple pulmonary metastasis of mouse osteosarcoma less than 1 mm of diameter, it is easily detected by fluorescence. We investigated sequential changes of AO fluorescence intensity from both of the mouse osteosarcoma tissue and muscles after AO injection. AO rapidly flew into both of the tumor and muscles, however muscles excluded AO quickly within 2 hours. On the other hand, the tumor slowly excluded AO, which still remained in the tumor even 2 hours later. Therefore, AO is retained in the tumor longer than in muscles [18, 21].

2. Selective Accumulation of AO in Human Musculoskeletal Sarcomas

Because the surgically resected tumor specimens emit intense green fluorescence from only the tumor and not from surrounding normal tissues after exposure to AO solution by ex vivo immersion followed by blue excitation, we have confirmed that most human malignant bone and soft tissue tumors are sensitive to AO staining [23].

Using those fresh sarcoma materials, we investigated the relationship between tumor acidity and AO fluorescence intensity. Average pH of resected tissues, measured using needle type pH meter was 6.78 in 35 sarcomas, 7.16 in 27 benign tumors, 7.26 in normal muscles and 7.43 in normal adipose tissues. Fluorescence intensity of AO increased in a manner dependent on acidity of those tissues. An acidic malignant tumor showed high AO fluorescence intensity. The result suggests that selective AO binding to musculoskeletal sarcomas is due to acidic extracellular fluid and acidic lysosome of sarcoma cells [23]. Staining with AO is therefore useful to visually detect tumor localization during surgery under fluorescence microscope, which makes it easy for surgeons to excise only tumor tissue with minimal damage of normal tissue (Photodynamic surgery: PDS) [18, 22].

3. Cytocidal Effect of AO-PDT on Osteosarcoma Cells

Results of our basic studies also revealed that AO had a strong cytocidal effect on mouse osteosarcoma cells after blue light illumination (AO-PDT), both in vitro and in vivo [16, 17]. Osteosarcoma cells in vitro died quickly within 24 hours after exposure to 1 µg/ml of AO followed by light illumination for 10 minutes with 10,000 luminescence (same as lux unit) and all cells completely died within 72 hours. Cells were swelled with cytoplasmic bleb formation and fragmented with microvesicle or exosome secretion, resulting in apoptosis. This cytocidal effect also occurred in multi-drug resistant osteosarcoma cells [16].

In vivo studies using a mouse osteosarcoma model, tumor growth was significantly inhibited by 10 mg/kg AO injection to intra-peritoneum followed by light illumination on tumor [17]. This result suggested that AO would be useful for photodynamic therapy in musculoskeletal sarcomas.

4. Cytocidal Effect of AO-RDT on Mouse Osteosarcoma Cells

Furthermore, we found that low-dose X-ray irradiation with 5 Gy of a mouse osteosarcoma after exposure to AO showed the same strong cytocidal effect in vitro and in vivo as that of AO-PDT [19]. This radiation effect with AO was proved by an Iowa University group in the USA in 2006 [30], independently of our group. They showed that AO exposure followed by X-ray irradiation with 3 Gy significantly enhanced cell death in radio-resistant chondrosarcoma cells, but not in radio-sensitive cells. Therefore, this effect might be mediated through a different mechanism from AO-PDT. However, it is a certain fact that AO enhances the radiation effect of killing cancer cells.

We have called this method radiodynamic therapy (RDT). X-ray irradiation has an advantage in reaching deeper areas of the human body than a light beam, even though it is more injurious to normal tissues. Indeed, AO itself also invades deeper tissues quickly at the rate of 5 mm per 30 minutes.

5. Mechanism of AO Accumulation and Cytocidal Effect of AO-PDT and AO-RDT in Osteosarcoma Cells

We investigated mechanisms of selective accumulation of AO in musculoskeletal sarcoma tissue. Many of recent papers have revealed that; 1) cancer cells produce a lot of proton (H^+) by active glycolysis under hypoxia or Warburg's effect [31, 32]; 2) proton is stored into lysosomes and acidic vesicles by Vocuolar-ATPase (V-ATPase), resulting in lysosomes and acid vesicles being more acidic in cancer cells than in normal cells [33, 34]; 3) the extracellular fluid around cancer cells is also more acidic due to more proton excluded from cytosolic space by NHE (Na- H^+ exchanger), V-APTase and

MCT (monocarboxylate transporter) than one of normal cells or produced by carbonic anhydrase 9 [35]. Since AO is accumulated into acidic environments, sarcoma cells having a lot of large acidic vesicles that are not able to exclude AO easily, whereas normal cells with non-acidic environments and weak acidic lysosomes can quickly exclude AO. It has been clarified that the inhibition of V-ATPase activity by bafilomycin causes a decrease in AO accumulation into the lysosome [23, 36], suggesting that AO accumulates into the lysosome in an acidity-dependent manner.

Therefore, our hypothesis on AO accumulation mechanism in sarcoma is as below. Active glycolysis through lactate produces a lot of hydrogen ions (proton) that are stored into lysosomes or acidic vesicles by V-ATPase. The extracellular fluid around cancer cells is also acidic due to the extrusion of protons by various proton transporters. Locally or systemically administered AO first accumulates into the acidic extracellular fluid and passively flows into cytosolic space followed by an accumulation into lysosomes depending on low pH (high acidity), and also accumulates into RNA by intercalation that is a different type of binding from that into lysosomes.

We also presume mechanisms of cytocidal effect of AO on sarcoma cells. AO accumulates into sarcoma cell lysosomes in an acidity-dependent manner. When photon energy of the blue light illuminates AO, AO is excited. Excited AO activates oxygen in lysosomes by emitting fluorescence, becoming a stable type of AO. Activated oxygen (singlet oxygen) oxidizes fatty acid of lysosomal membrane, resulting in leakage of various lysosomal enzymes such as protease, lipase and nuclease into cytosolic space. It has been reported that a singlet oxygen scavenger like L-histidine inhibits a cytocidal effect of AO-PDT [16, 36]. A lot of protons also leak into the cytosolic space, which becomes acidic. Those enzymes digest important cell components under an acidic cytosolic condition. Such lysosomal stress activates caspase, causing cellular apoptosis with cell swelling, bleb formation, release of microparticles including exosomes and cellular fragmentation.

6. Inhibitory Effect of AO-PDT on Local Recurrence after Intra-Lesional Tumor Excision of Mouse Osteosarcoma Model

Before the clinical application of AO-PDT to human sarcomas, we performed a simulation study of curettage (intralesional tumor excision) supported by AO-PDT, using a mouse model. AO of 10 mg/kg was intraperitoneally injected to mice with a tumor at the back. After 2 hours, the tumor was surgically curetted followed by additional microscopic curettage under fluorovisualization with blue light illumination using fluorescence surgical microscope. Finally, blue light was illuminated on the tumor-resected area for 10 minutes (AO-PDT). The results showed that AO-PDT after macroscopic and microscopic curettage of a mouse osteosarcoma significantly inhibited local tumor recurrence. The recurrence rate was 80% in the control group, while it was 23% in the treated group receiving AO-PDT [18].

Clinical Application of AOT to Patients

1. Procedure of AOT

The procedure for clinical application of AOT is that 1) macroscopic curettage of tumor is first performed; 2) additional microscopic curettage with ultrasonic surgical knife under tumor visualization with green fluorescence is performed after local administration of 1μg/ml AO solution for 5 minutes followed by excitation with blue light using fluorescence surgical microscope (PDS); 3) consequently, AO-PDT is applied to tumor curettage area for 10 minutes using surgical microscope; 4) after closure of surgical wound without washing-out of AO solution, 5 Gy of X-ray is immediately irradiated to the resected area for AO-RDT [23-28] (Figure 1).

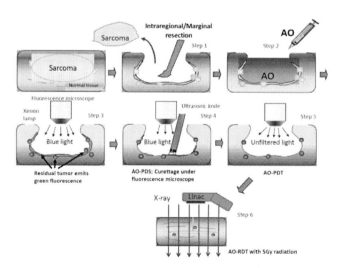

Figure 1. Surgical procedure of AOT (AO-PDS, AO-PDT and AO-RDT).

Table 1. Histological Diagnosis, Location and AJCC Staging

	Histological diagnosis		Location		AJCC staging	
Soft tissue sarcoma (51)	Synovial Sarcoma	9	Thigh	13	II	13
	MFH	8	Forearm	8	III	25
	Rhabdomyosarcoma	7	Buttock	6	IV	13
	Leiomyosarcoma	6	Knee	5		
	Extraskeletal myxoid chondorosarcoma	4	Trunk	5		
	PNET	4	Lower leg	4		
	Fibrosarcoma	4	Foot	3		
	Liposarcoma	4	Inguinal region	2		
	Sclerosing epithelioid fibrasarcoma	1	Upper arm	2		
	Synovial Chondrosarcoma	1	Shoulder	2		
	Neuroblastoma	1	Hand	1		
	Alveolar soft part sarcoma	1				
	Epithelioid sarcoma	1				

Table 2. Histological Diagnosis, Location and AJCC Staging

	Histological diagnosis		Location		AJCC staging	
Bone Sarcoma (16)	Osteosarcoma	8	Humerus	5	I	2
	Ewing Sarcoma	4	Femur	4	II	10
	Chondrosarcoma	4	Ilium	2	IV	4
			Radius	2		
			Tibia	1		
			Fibula	1		
			Rib/ Vertebral body	1		

2. Patients

We have applied AOT to 67 patients with high grade malignant musculoskeletal sarcomas under control of IRB of our hospitals with agreement with patients and closed families after full explanation of the clinical study. The 51 soft tissue sarcoma patients included high grade malignant sarcomas such as synovial sarcomas, rhabdomyosarcomas, MHFs, leiomyosarcomas, etc. (Table. 1) and 15 bone sarcoma patients also included high grade malignant sarcomas such as osteosarcomas and Ewing's sarcomas (Table 2).

3. Clinical Outcome

Clinical outcome showed that the 5-year survival rate (SR) was 67.8 % and the 5-year local recurrence-free rate (LRFR) was and 71.2 % in all of 57 patients with soft-tissue sarcoma. In AJCC classification, SR was 100% in stage II, 86.7 % in stage III and 0 % in stage IV, and LRFR was 92.3% in stage II, 64.3 % in stage III and 60.2 % in stage IV. In tumor size classification, LRFR was 78% in smaller tumors than 10 cm, while 46.2% in larger tumors (Figure 2).

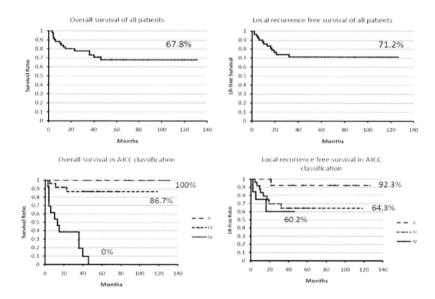

Figure 2. Overall survival rate and local recurrence- free rate in patients with malignant soft tissue tumor.

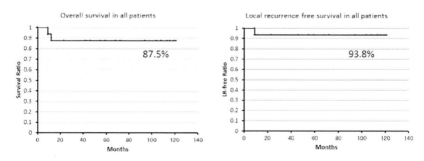

Figure 3. Overall survival rate and local recurrence-free rate in patients with malignant bone tumors.

On the other hand, SR was 85.7 % and the LRFR was and 93.8 % in all of the 15 cases of high-grade malignant bone sarcoma (Figure 3). The local control rate of AO-PDT is not superior to that of conventional wide resection surgery, but its limb function after surgery is far superior. Most patients had an excellent limb function as running fast, jumping, swimming and throwing ball well.

We believe that all of our patients in this study might spend the rest of their lives as mostly normal or not handicapped people. To keep such good limb function is very important for sarcoma survivors, especially in children in order to keep long high quality of life after surgery.

Toxicity and Carcinogenicity of AO

People believe that because AO is mutagen of bacteria [37, 38], it would be a carcinogen for human. However, this is not true. Although there were some reports to investigate carcinogenicity of AO [39, 40], no one has any evidence of AO carcinogenesis. Therefore, the International Agency of Research on Cancer (IARC) of WHO or other official reports do not classify AO as a carcinogen [41]. We know some reports on the application of AO to human clinical studies in addition to ours. Two Japanese papers have reported to use AO for diagnosis of cervical cancer or gastric cancer by local or oral administration [42, another in Japanese]. Recently, a study reported by Italian group has applied our method of AO-RDT for one synovial sarcoma patient [43]. In 2009, a USA group has also applied AO to some patients with ovarian disease in clinical study of confocal laser laparoscopic biopsy under a condition with FDA approval [44]. The FDA in the USA has approved application of AO in particular clinical study after investigation of acute and chronic toxicity and carcinogenicity using mice [45]. Our study using mice revealed that LD_{50} of AO intravenously administrated was 28-30mg/kg [21]. Those clinical reports have not shown any serious complication caused by AO administration. Since the concentration of AO solution used by us in the clinical study was very low, and AO was administered only locally, we believe that the risk of carcinogenesis induced by AO in our patients was significantly lower than that by most other known anti-cancer agents.

Conclusion

In conclusion, based on basic research and clinical data, we strongly believe that AOT consisting of AO-PDS, AO-PDT and AO-RDT may be a promising new limb salvage modality for the preservation of excellent limb function with low risk of local tumor recurrence in musculoskeletal sarcoma patients, and may also be applicable to many other solid cancers, although studies on a larger number of patients with longer durations of follow-up are required.

References

[1] Mangat KS, Jeys LM, Carter SR. Latest developments in limb-salvage surgery in osteosarcoma. *Exper. Rev. Anti-cancer Ther.* 2011; 11: 205-15.

[2] Steinau H-U, Daigeler AD, Langer S, Steinstrasser L, Hauser J, Goertz O, Lehnhardt M. Limb salvage in Malignant Tumors. *Semin. Plast Surg.* 2010; 24: 18-33.

[3] Aksnes LH, Bauer HC, Jebsen NL, Folleras G, Allert C, Haugen GS, Hall KS. Limb-sparing surgery preserves more function than amputation: a Scandiavian sarcoma group study of 118 patients. *J. Bone Joint Surg. Br.* 2008; 90: 786-94.

[4] Tunn PU, Pomraenke D, Goerling U, Hohenberger P. Functional outcome after endoprosthetic limb-salvage therapy of primary bone tumors – a comparative analysis using the MSTS scoe, the TESS and RNL index. *International Orthopaedics* 2008; 32: 619-25.

[5] Abed R, Grimer R. Surgical modalities in the treatment of bone sarcoma in children. *Cancer Treatment Reviews* 2010; 36: 324-47.

[6] Bekkering WP, Vlieland TPMV, Koopman HM, Schaap GR, Schireuder HWB, Beishuizen A, Jutte PC, Hoogerbrugge PH, Anninga JK, Nelissen RGHH, Taminiau AHM. Functional ability and physical activity in children and young adults after limb-salvage or ablative surgery for lower extremity bone tumors. *J. Surg. Oncol.* 2010;103: 276-82.

[7] Kapuscinski J, Darzynkiewicz Z and Melamed MR. Interactions of acridine orange with nucleic acids. Properties of complexes of acridine orange with single stranded ribonucleic acid. *Biochem. Pharmacol.* 1983; 32: 3679-94.

[8] Amagasa J. Mechanisms of photodynamic inactivation of acridine orange-sensitized transfer RNA: participation of singlet oxygen and base damage leading to inactivation. *J. Radiat. Res.* (Tokyo) 1986; 27: 339-51.

[9] Cools AA, Jansen LHM: Fluorescence response of acridine orange to changes in pH gradients across liposome membranes. *Experimentia* 1986; 42: 954-956

[10] Zdolsek JM, Olsson GM and Brunk UT. Photooxidative damage to lysosomes of cultured macrophages by acridine orange. *Photochem. Photobiol.* 1990; 51: 67-76.

[11] Sastry KS and Gordon MP. The photodynamic inactivation of tobacco mosaic virus and its ribonucleic acid by acridine orange. *Biochim. Biophys. Acta* 1966; 129: 32-41.

[12] Lewis RM and Goland PP. In vivo staining and retardation of tumors in mice by acridine compounds. *Am. J. Med. Sci.* 1948; 215: 282-9.

[13] Korgaonkar K and Sukhatankara J. Anti-tumor activity of the fluorescent dye, acridine orange, on Yoshida sarcoma (ascites). *Br. J. Cancer* 1963; 17: 471-3.

[14] Giorgio A, Rambaldi M, Maccario P, Ambrosone L and Moles DA. Detection of microorganisms in clinical specimens using slides pre-stained with acridine orange (AOS). *Microbiologica* 1989; 12: 97-100.

[15] Rickman L, Long G, Oberst R, Cabanban A, Sangalang R, Smith J, Chulay J and Hoffman S. Rapid diagnosis of malaria by acridine orange staining of centrifuged parasites. *Lancet* 1989; 14: 68-71.

[16] Kusuzaki K, Minami G, Takeshita H, Murata H, Hashiguchi S, Nozaki T, Ashihara T and Hirasawa Y. Photodynamic inactivation with acridine orange on a multi-drug-resistant mouse osteosarcoma cell line. *Jpn. J. Cancer Res.* 2000; 91: 439-45.

[17] Kusuzaki K, Aomori, K, Suginoshita, Minami G, Takeshita H, Murata H, Hashiguchi S, Ashihara T and Hirasawa Y. Total tumor cell elimination with minimum damage to normal tissues in musculoskeletal sarcomas by photodynamic reaction with acridine orange. *Oncology-Bazel.* 2000; 59: 174-80.

[18] Kusuzaki K, Suginoshita T, Minami G, Aomori K, Takeshita H, Murata H, Hashiguchi S, Ashihara T and Hirasawa Y. Fluorovisualization effect of acridine orange on mouse osteosarcoma. *Anticancer Res.* 2000; 20: 3019-24.

[19] Hashiguchi S, Kusuzaki K, Murata H, Takeshita H, Hashiba M, Nishimura T, Ashihara T and Hirasawa Y: Acridine orange excited by

low-dose radiation has a strong cytocidal effect on mouse osteosarcoma. *Oncology-Bazel* 2002; 62: 85-93.

[20] Kusuzaki K, Murata H, Takeshita H, Hashiguchi S, Nozaki T, Emoto K, Ashihara T and Hirasawa Y. Intracellular binding sites of acridine orange in living osteosarcoma cells. *Anticancer Res.* 2000; 20:971-6.

[21] Satonaka H, Kusuzaki K, Shintani K, Matsumine A, Matsubara T, Wakabayashi T, Uchida A. Extracorporeal photodynamic image detection of mouse osteosarcoma in soft tissues utilizing fluorovisualization effect of acridine orange. *Oncology (Bazel)* 2007; 70:465-73.

[22] Matsubara T, Kusuzaki K, Matsumine A, Shintani K, Satonaka H and Uchida A . Acridine orange used for photodynamic therapy accumulates in malignant musculoskeletal tumors depending on pH gradient. *Anticancer Res.* 2006; 26: 187-94.

[23] Kusuzaki K, Murata H, Matsubara T, Miyazaki S, Okamura A, Seto M, Matsumine A, Hosoi H, Sugimoto T and Uchida A : Clinical outcome of a new photodynamic therapy with acridine orange for synovial sarcomas. *Photochem. Photobiol.* 81: 705-9, 2005.

[24] Kusuzaki K, Murata H, Matsubara T, Miyazaki S, Okamura A, Seto M, Matsumine A, Hosoi H, Sugimoto T and Uchida A: Clinical trial of photodynamic therapy using acridine orange with/without low dose radiation as new limb salvage modality in musculoskeletal sarcomas. *Anti-cancer Res.* 2005; 25: 1225-36.

[25] Nakamura T, Kusuzaki K, Matsubara T, Matsumine A, Murata H, Uchida A. A new limb salvage surgery in cases of high-grade soft tissue sarcoma using photodynamic surgery, followed by photo- and radio-dynamic therapy with acridine orange. *J. Surg. Oncol.* 2008; 97: 523-8.

[26] Matsubara T, Kusuzaki K, Matsumine A, Murata H, Satonaka H, Shinntani K, Nakamura T, Hosoi H, Iehara T, Sugimoto T, Uchida A. A new therapeutic modality involving acridine orange excitation by photon energy used during reduction surgery for rhabodomyosarcomas. *Oncol. Rep.* 2009; 21: 89-94.

[27] Matsubara T, Kusuzaki K, Matsumine A, Murata H, Nakamura T, Uchida A, Sudo A. Clinical outcomes of minimally invasive surgery using acridine orange for musculoskeletal sarcomas around the forearm, compared with conventional limb salvage surgery after wide resection. *J. Surg. Oncol.* 2010; 102: 271-5.

[28] Matsubara T, Kusuzaki K, Matsumine A, Murata H, Marunaka Y, Hosogi S, Uchida A, Sudo A. Photodynamic therapy with acridine

orangein musculoskeletal sarcomas. *J. Bone Joint Surg. (Br.)* 2010; 92: 760-2.
[29] Zelenin AV. Fluorescence microscopy of lysosomes and related structures in living cells. *Nature* 1966; 212: 425-6.
[30] Moussavi-Harami F, Mollano A, Martin JA, Ayoob A, Domann FE, Gitelis S and Buckwalter JA . Intrinsic radiation resistance in human chondrosarcoma. *BBRC* 2006; 346: 379-85.
[31] Gatenby RA, Gillies RJ: Why do cancers have high aerobic glycolysis? *Nature Review* 2004; 4: 891-890.
[32] Yamagata M, Hasuda K, Stamato T, Tannock IF: The contribution of lactic acid to acidification of tumors: studies of variant cells lacking lactate dehydrogenase. *Br. J. Cancer* 1998; 77: 1726-1731.
[33] De Milito A, Canese R, Marino ML, Borghi M, Iero M, Villa A, Venturi G, Lozupone F, Iessi E, Logozzi M, Della Mina P, Santinami M, Rodolfo M, Podo F, Rivoltini L, Fais S: pH-dependent anti-tumor activity of proton pump inhibitors against human melanoma is mediated by inhibition of tumor acidity. *Int. J. Cancer* 2010 127: 207-219.
[34] Fais S, De Milito A, You H, You H, Qin W: Targeting vacuolar H+-ATPase as a new strategy against cancer. *Cancer Res.* 2007; 67: 10627-10630.
[35] Swietach P, Vaughan-Jones RD, Harris AL. *Regulation of tumor pH and the role of carbonic anhyrase* 9. 2007; 26: 299-310.
[36] Hiruma H, Katakura T, Igawa S, Kanoh M, Fujimura T, Kawakami T. Vesicle disruption, plasma membrane bleb formation, and acute cell death caused by illumination with blue light in acridine orange-loaded malignant melanoma cells. *J. Photochem. Photobiol.* B 2007; 86: 1-8.
[37] Zampieri A and Greenberg J. Mutagenesis by acridine orange and proflavin in Escherichia coli strain S. *Mutat. Res.* 1965; 2: 552-6.
[38] McCann J, Choi E, Yamasaki E and Ames BN. Detection of carcinogenesis as mutagens in the Salmonella/microsome test: Assay of 300 chemicals. *Proc. Natl. Acad. Sci. USA* 1975; 72: 5135-9.
[39] Van Duuren, Sivak A, Katz C, Melchionne S. Tumorigenecity of acridine orange. *Br. J. Cancer* 1969; 23: 587-90.
[40] Beeken WL, Roessner KD. In vivo labeling of hepatic lysosomes by intragastric administration of acridine orange. *Lab. Invest.* 1972; 26: 173-77
[41] International Agency for Research on Cancer. Acridine Orange. In: *IARC Monographs Program on the Evaluation of Carcinogenic Risks to Human.* IARC Press Lyon, 1978;16:145

[42] Kato A. Gastrofiberscopic diagnosis with acridie orange fluorescence. *Gastroenterol. Endosc.* 1970;12: 351-62.

[43] Coli A, et al: Myxoid monophasic synovial sarcoma: case report of an unusual histological variant. *J. Exp. Clin. Cancer Res.* 2006; 25: 287-91.

[44] Tanbakuchi AA, Rouse AR, Udovich JA, Hatch KD, Gmitro AF. In vivo imaging of ovarian tissue using a novel confocal microlaparoscope. *J. Biomed. Optics* 2009; 14: 044030.

[45] Udovich JA, Besselsen DG, Gmitro AF. Assessment of acridine orange and SYTO 16 for in vivo imaging of the peritoneal tissues in mice. *J. Microscopy* 2009; 234: 124-9.

In: Sarcoma
Editor: Eric J. Butler

ISBN: 978-1-62100-362-5
© 2012 Nova Science Publishers, Inc.

Chapter VII

The Role of Surgery in Children with Head and Neck Rhabdomyosarcoma and Ewing's Sarcoma

P. Gradoni, D. Giordano, G. Oretti,
M. Fantoni and T. Ferri
Department of Otorhinolaryngology,
University of Parma, Parma, Italy

Introduction

Rhabdomyosarcoma (RMS) is a soft tissue malignant neoplasm and it is the most common paediatric solid tumour [1]. Ewing's sarcoma (ES) is a primary bone malignant neoplasm and it is the second most common primary malignant tumour of bone found in children after osteosarcoma [2]. These tumours are uncommon in adults: RMS follows a bimodal distribution, with peak incidence between 2 and 4 years and between 12 and 16 years [3]. Ewing's sarcoma has a peak incidence during the second decade of life [4]. Head and neck localizations are frequent in RMS, accounting for 35-40% of the cases while they are rare in ES (1-4%) [1,2,5].

Rhabdomyosarcoma and ES share some crucial biologic and clinical features: they are high grade tumours with local aggressiveness and strong potential to metastasize; both tumours are considered "systemic diseases" given the rapid development of metastatic spread. Because of that, systemic chemotherapy plays an essential role in treating distant metastases regardless their identification at initial staging [1,4]; unlike other soft tissue sarcomas and osteogenic sarcoma, RMS and ES are relatively sensitive to chemotherapy and radiotherapy [3]; in other sarcomas there are no good alternative to radical surgery [6]; standard treatment for RMS and ES is a multimodal therapy involving chemotherapy, radiotherapy and surgery [7,8]; until 1991, patients with extraosseous ES were eligible for the Intergroup Rhabdomyosarcoma Study (IRS) protocols [9].

Prior to the introduction of antineoplastic drugs, surgery played the central role in the cure of patients with RMS and ES [4,10]; in the last four decades, the development of multi-agent chemotherapy protocols resulted in a significant improvement in long-term survival: from 25% (RMS) and 10% (ES) in 1970, to approximately 70% nowadays [4,10]. Such scenario has leaded to a critical discussion in literature concerning the role of surgical treatment. Particular surgical challenge is represented by tumours affecting the head and neck. These anatomical sites do not generally lend themselves to a radical surgical approach as a primary procedure [7]; complete resection is not feasible in many patients and, even if possible, is unlikely to be achieved without major functional or cosmetic consequences [7]. Nevertheless, radical surgery is still considered the best choice to obtain the local control [1,4]. Very few studies have been focused on the feasibility and effectiveness of surgical resection [11]. Defined criteria to establish the risks and the benefits of surgical treatment do not exist at this time [8]. Despite the improvement in diagnostic techniques, especially imaging, some authors acknowledge that incomplete surgical excision may be due to inadequate preoperative evaluation [3,12]. Given the rarity of these neoplasms, most studies deal with relatively small surgical series or even case reports; indications evidently arise from personal experiences and many authors conclude that the surgical treatment should be decided on a case by case basis [13].

In order to delineate the role of surgery in head and neck RMS and ES, indications, feasibility and timing criteria of surgical treatment have been reviewed and extracted from literature. The management of orbital RMS is unique because surgery does not confer any advantage over chemotherapy and radiotherapy in terms of survival [14,15], thus it won't be discussed herein.

Biopsy

Diagnosis always requires a biopsy [4,11]. Authors widely agree that open biopsy is to be preferred [3,4,10,12,16-21].

Rhabdomyosarcoma

Open surgical biopsy represents the recommended technique since it allows to obtain an adequate specimen for pathological, biological and treatment protocol studies. Superficial and accessible lesions or lesions with inconclusive results from prior closed biopsy should be biopsied by incisional or excisional technique. Endoscopic techniques play a key role in exploring and specimen sampling the sinonasal sarcomas [20]. Closed techniques such as fine needle aspiration and core needle biopsy, by obtaining smaller volume of tissue, increase sampling error and inconclusive findings and may preclude molecular biology studies [22]. Fine needle aspiration or core needle biopsy should be reserved for deeper and less accessible lesions [10], metastatic disease or small lesions in areas that will be treated primarily by chemotherapy and radiotherapy [3].

Ewing's Sarcoma

Diagnosis should be achieved by means of core needle or surgical biopsy[23].

Debulking Surgery

Debulking surgery consists in a partial tumour resection with macroscopic residuals [12].

Rhabdomyosarcoma

There are no evidences that debulking operations offer advantages with regard to patient outcome. Debulking surgery is considered a practicable choice in urgent situation or as a palliative intervention to improve the appearance or to eliminate the offensive odor from necrotic tumour in patients with uncontrolled disease [12,14,20].

Ewing's Sarcoma

Similarly, debulking surgery in Ewing's sarcoma does not seem to offer any advantages in terms of local control, and its role appears to be limited to palliative aims [4,24].

Radical Surgery as Primary Treatment Modality

Rhabdomyosarcoma

Radical surgery as primary treatment modality should be always taken into consideration in RMS. Complete surgical resection with negative margins offers the best chance of controlling local disease [1,14]. Survival clearly depends on the amount of residual disease after surgery [15,25] so that complete tumour resection is recommended whenever locoregional removal appears possible [3,11,13,26]. Moreover, a complete resection with negative margins in favourable sites (i.e. non-parameningeal) permits to avoid radiotherapy and its late toxicity [1,7,14]. Complete resection of the primary tumour has to include a surrounding "envelope" of normal tissue [3]. However, has to be remarked that in head and neck localizations, radical resection, when feasible, usually implies major functional and cosmetic consequences [1,3,7]. Most author discourage primary surgery when it may lead to unacceptable morbidity [7,12,13,21]. Orbit exenteratio, cranial nerves sacrifice, resection of vital structures such as the larynx and pharynx, demolitive procedures towards bones and soft tissues of the head and neck with poor reconstructive options are cited as major consequences of radical surgery [12,14,27]. Tumours limited to soft tissue may not be well delineated and are difficult to clinically and radiologically distinguish from surrounding inflammatory reaction. Thus the accurate assessment of the extent of tumour and its resecability is often possible only at the time of surgery [14].

In the head and neck area, a distinction is drawn between parameningeal RMS (PM-RMS) and RMS of other localizations. Parameningeal RMS arises at sites with a particularly close anatomic relationship with the meninges such as nasopharynx, nasal cavity, paranasal sinuses, middle ear and mastoid, infratemporal and pterygopalatine fossa. They represents a particular surgical challenge. Surgical excision may lead to unacceptable mutilations and incomplete resection in most cases [28]. These tumours have a high likelihood of meningeal extension, which is considered a fatal pattern of progression [9,29,30]. Cranial nerve palsy, skull base invasion and intracranial extension have been considered the high-risk features for meningeal involvement [9,21]. Meningeal involvement is an independent negative prognostic factor and a significant predictor of primary central nervous system failure [9].

The introduction of systematic radiotherapy has improved survival for children with PM-RMS, and cure of these patients remains difficult without this element of treatment; thus, even a complete surgical resection with negative margins may not avoid radiotherapy [7,9,14,21,29].

These issues lead most authors to conclude that multi-agent chemotherapy combined with radiation is the primary treatment modality offered to children with PM-RMS [3,7,11,14,28]. Surgery prior to cytoreductive chemotherapy is recommended if there is no intracranial extension, if complete resection seems feasible and if it won't lead to unacceptable morbidity [11,14,26,31].

Nowadays, complete imaging investigation with computed tomography and magnetic resonance scanning allows to define the precise extent of the tumour as well as the presence of high-risk features of meningeal involvement, so that a more appropriate treatment plan can be stated.

When primary excision leaves positive margins, primary pretreatment re-excision may be useful [10]. Primary pretreatment re-excision refers to an operative procedure that consists in a wide excision of the previous operative site, including an adequate margin of normal tissue with careful examination of all margins before adjuvant therapy [3]. Many authors consider this measure as advisable in certain circumstances or even necessary when radiotherapy is to be avoided [3,10,11,14]. Complete tumour removal improves survival and offers the chance to avoid radiotherapy, which is of special interest in children younger than 3 years old [10,32,33]. This revision surgery should be performed with frozen-section control of the margins. Evidently the feasibility criteria follow those mentioned for primary resection [14].

Ewing's Sarcoma

Radical surgery is not provided as primary treatment modality. The current standard treatment of Ewing's sarcoma begins with chemotherapy, unless otherwise contraindicated. Even when the tumour appears resectable, patients are submitted to 4-6 cycles of neoadjuvant chemotherapy to eradicate micrometastatic disease and facilitate effective local control measures with wide negative margins [1,2,4,8,23,34].

Surgery after Primary Chemoradiation

Chemotherapy and radiotherapy have proven capable of shrinking, and even eradicating, primary tumours. Clinical and radiological re-staging to evaluate surgical indications has to be part of the treatment strategy [1,3,7,10,11,14,31,32,35].

Rhabdomyosarcoma

Surgery after primary chemoradiation has been called "second look operation (SLO)"; the purpose of SLO was firstly to determine pathologic response and to remove residual tumour to achieve local control [3]. Currently, authors agree that SLO is unreliable in establishing true complete pathological response in patients with a clinical response [7,10,36,37]. Second look operation in order to remove residual tumour is strongly recommended because of its efficacy in reducing the local relapse rate [3,7,10,14]. In PM-RMS, as discussed above, surgery is mainly performed after primary adjuvant treatment [7,11,20].

Ewing's Sarcoma

Surgery after chemotherapy is the current standard of cure [2,8,23,34]. Despite the lack of randomized trials comparing different local treatment modalities in ES, wide surgical resection is considered the treatment of choice. It reduces the local relapse rate, improves the overall survival and may avoid radiotherapy [4-6,24,38,39]. It is commonly accepted that an attempt at complete tumour resection should always be made [6,39]. Nevertheless chemoradiation may be a reasonable alternative to surgery for treatment of tumours that are resectable only with an unacceptable degree of mutilation [2,6,40].

Lymphnode Dissection

Rhabdomyosarcoma

Head and neck RMS has proven able to spread to cervical lymphnodes. Comparing the two most frequent histologic subtypes i.e. embryonal and alveolar, the latter showed a statistically significant higher tendency to metastasize through the lymphatic route [13]. Most authors recommend elective neck dissection for therapeutic and staging purposes in patients with alveolar RMS when surgery on primary tumour is planned [13]. Clinically positive nodes should always be confirmed pathologically and core needle biopsy or fine needle aspiration are appropriate [3]. Controversy exists also over treating the N+ neck with additional radiotherapy or neck dissection [11]. If nodes are metastatic and complete primary tumour resection is feasible, neck dissection is recommended [11]; while, if the lymphnodes are positive but the primary tumour is unresectable, they should be included in the radiotherapy field [11].

Ewing's Sarcoma

Lymphnodes metastasis from Ewing's sarcoma are very rare [4]. The nodal status included as a prognostic indicator in the American Joint Committee on Cancer (AJCC) staging system has even been considered irrelevant by some authors [8]. Considering this, it can be argued that elective neck dissection is not indicated. Nevertheless, this argument is not discussed in the literature.

Salvage Surgery after Locoregional Relapse

Rhabdomyosarcoma

The survival rate after relapse is a dismal 10-15%[46]. Various therapeutic efforts have been attempted including surgical resection, radical neck dissection, thoracotomy, laminectomy and tumour embolization, but results were poor. Second-line chemotherapy and radiotherapy are the main treatment options in presence of relapsing disease. Although surgery is advocated for resectable recurrent tumour, the evidence for its efficacy is very limited [28,44,47,48].

Ewing's Sarcoma

Also in ES relapsing disease has an awful 5-years survival rate (i.e. <10%) [49]. Nevertheless, selected patients with solitary lesions may benefit from aggressive salvage treatment [8,49]. In particular, late relapses may be treated with curative intent and have a better prognosis than early ones [34,39].

Metastasectomy

Rhabdomyosarcoma

The outcome for patients with metastatic RMS is especially poor[7]. Surgery has a limited role in the patient with metastatic disease [10]; a retrospective study by Temeck et al evaluating the outcome of pulmonary metastasis resection found a poor result among patient with RMS [50]. If a resectable pulmonary nodule remains after chemotherapy or radiotherapy, excision might be considered since there may be little else to offer these patients that affords any better prospects [10].

Ewing's Sarcoma

Patients with metastatic disease are offered chemoradiation [2]. On rare occasions, limited pulmonary metastases can be resected but the 5-year survival for those with metastatic disease remains approximately 25% [8].

Conclusions

Together with chemotherapy and radiotherapy, surgery plays a pivotal role in the treatment of head and neck RMS and ES. Diagnosis has to be achieved by a surgical biopsy, whereas closed techniques should be adopted only in case of inaccessible lesions. Debulking surgery does not offer any advantage in term of curative results, while can be considered for palliative purposes.

Great improvement in survival has been made during the past 40 years especially for patients with localized disease, while prognosis for patients with metastatic or recurrent disease remains poor. Therefore, an effective and timely local control of disease has a key role in the management of these tumours. Despite the optimal modality for local control remains controversial, surgery is advocated as the treatment of choice. Staging work-up by means of high resolution computed tomography and magnetic resonance imaging of the head and neck provides essential preoperative information. Tumour relationship with skull base and meninges represents a major aspect in evaluating surgical indication, relapsing rate and overall prognosis. Elective neck dissection is recommended in alveolar RMS when surgery on primary tumour is planned.

Progress in the fields of skull base surgery, microsurgery and plastic-reconstructive surgery, offers nowadays the option of reconstructing important structures with functionally and cosmetically satisfactory results. Nonetheless, demolitive surgery in children with head and neck tumours may lead to unacceptable consequences. This is a common scenario in head and neck regions and frequently the harm/benefit ratio tends in favour of chemoradiation.

Appropriate indications and timing of the surgical treatment are of paramount importance to offer the best chance of survival and the lower morbidity. Clear and widely shared surgical criteria should be advisable so that a correct and precise preoperative plan can be stated. Multidisciplinary team including oncologists, radiotherapists, ENT surgeons, neurosurgeons and maxillofacial surgeons is required in the management of these tumours.

References

[46] Skubitz KM, D'Adamo DR. Sarcoma. *Mayo. Clin. Proc.* 2007 Nov;82(11):1409-32.
[47] Vaccani JP, Forte V, de Jong AL, Taylor G. Ewing's sarcoma of the head and neck in children. *Int. J. Pediatr. Otorhinolaryngol.* 1999 May 25;48(3):209-16.
[48] Rodeberg DA, Paidas CN, Lobe TL, et al. Surgical Principles for Children/Adolescents With Newly Diagnosed Rhabdomyosarcoma: A Report from the Soft Tissue Sarcoma Committee of the Children's Oncology Group. *Sarcoma* 2002;6(4):111-22.
[49] Iwamoto Y. Diagnosis and treatment of Ewing's sarcoma. *Jpn. J. Clin. Oncol.* 2007 Feb;37(2):79-89.
[50] Siegal GP, Oliver WR, Reinus WR, et al. Primary Ewing's sarcoma involving the bones of the head and neck. *Cancer* 1987 Dec 1;60(11):2829-40.
[51] Daw NC, Mahmoud HH, Meyer WH, et al. Bone sarcomas of the head and neck in children: the St Jude Children's Research Hospital experience. *Cancer* 2000 May 1;88(9):2172-80.
[52] Stevens MC. Treatment for childhood rhabdomyosarcoma: the cost of cure. *Lancet Oncol.* 2005 Feb;6(2):77-84.
[53] Ludwig JA. Ewing sarcoma: historical perspectives, current state-of-the-art, and opportunities for targeted therapy in the future. *Curr. Opin. Oncol.* 2008 Jul;20(4):412-8.
[54] Raney RB, Meza J, Anderson JR, et al. Treatment of children and adolescents with localized parameningeal sarcoma: experience of the Intergroup Rhabdomyosarcoma Study Group protocols IRS-II through -IV, 1978-1997. *Med. Pediatr. Oncol.* 2002 Jan;38(1):22-32.
[55] Schalow EL, Broecker BH. Role of surgery in children with rhabdomyosarcoma. *Med. Pediatr. Oncol.* 2003 Jul;41(1):1-6.
[56] Fyrmpas G, Wurm J, Athanassiadou F, et al. Management of paediatric sinonasal rhabdomyosarcoma. *J. Laryngol. Otol.* 2009 Sep;123(9):990-6.

[57] Cecchetto G, Bisogno G, De Corti F, et al. Biopsy or debulking surgery as initial surgery for locally advanced rhabdomyosarcomas in children?: the experience of the Italian Cooperative Group studies. *Cancer* 2007 Dec 1;110(11):2561-7.

[58] Wurm J, Constantinidis J, Grabenbauer GG, Iro H. Rhabdomyosarcomas of the nose and paranasal sinuses: treatment results in 15 cases. *Otolaryngol. Head Neck Surg.* 2005 Jul;133(1):42-50.

[59] Daya H, Chan HS, Sirkin W, Forte V. Pediatric rhabdomyosarcoma of the head and neck: is there a place for surgical management? *Arch. Otolaryngol. Head Neck Surg.* 2000 Apr;126(4):468-72.

[60] Maurer HM, Beltangady M, Gehan EA, et al. The Intergroup Rhabdomyosarcoma Study-I. A final report. *Cancer* 1988 Jan 15;61(2):209-20.

[61] Willman JH, White K, Coffin CM. Pediatric core needle biopsy: strengths and limitations in evaluation of masses. *Pediatr. Dev. Pathol.* 2001 Jan-Feb;4(1):46-52.

[62] Pohar-Marinsek Z, Anzic J, Jereb B. Topical topic: value of fine needle aspiration biopsy in childhood rhabdomyosarcoma: twenty-six years of experience in Slovenia. *Med. Pediatr. Oncol.* 2002 Jun;38(6):416-20.

[63] Kilpatrick SE, Cappellari JO, Bos GD, Gold SH, Ward WG. Is fine-needle aspiration biopsy a practical alternative to open biopsy for the primary diagnosis of sarcoma? Experience with 140 patients. *Am. J. Clin. Pathol.* 2001 Jan;115(1):59-68.

[64] Ahmed AA, Tsokos M. Sinonasal rhabdomyosarcoma in children and young adults. *Int. J. Surg. Pathol.* 2007 Apr;15(2):160-5.

[65] Herrmann BW, Sotelo-Avila C, Eisenbeis JF. Pediatric sinonasal rhabdomyosarcoma: three cases and a review of the literature. *Am. J. Otolaryngol.* 2003 May-Jun;24(3):174-80.

[66] Stevens MC, Rey A, Bouvet N, et al. Treatment of nonmetastatic rhabdomyosarcoma in childhood and adolescence: third study of the International Society of Paediatric Oncology –SIOP- Malignant Mesenchymal Tumor 89. *J. Clin. Oncol.* 2005 Apr 20;23(12):2618-28.

[67] Lietman S. Current management of soft tissue sarcomas *Curr. Opin. Orthop.* 2001 Dec12(6):505-508.

[68] www.nccn.org.

[69] Schuck A, Ahrens S, Paulussen M, et al. Local therapy in localized Ewing tumors: results of 1058 patients treated in the CESS 81, CESS 86, and EICESS 92 trials. *Int. J. Radiat. Oncol. Biol. Phys.* 2003 Jan 1;55(1):168-77.

[70] Wharam MD, Beltangady MS, Heyn RM, et al. Pediatric orofacial and laryngopharyngeal rhabdomyosarcoma. An Intergroup Rhabdomyosarcoma Study report. *Arch. Otolaryngol. Head Neck Surg.* 1987 Nov;113(11):1225-7.

[71] Healy GB, Upton J, Black PM, Ferraro N. The role of surgery in rhabdomyosarcoma of the head and neck in children. *Arch. Otolaryngol. Head Neck Surg.* 1991 Oct;117(10):1185-8.

[72] Anderson GJ, Tom LW, Womer RB, Handler SD, Wetmore RF, Potsic WP. Rhabdomyosarcoma of the head and neck in children. *Arch. Otolaryngol. Head Neck Surg.* 1990 Apr;116(4):428-31.

[73] Sercarz JA, Mark RJ, Tran L, Storper I, Calcaterra TC. Sarcomas of the nasal cavity and paranasal sinuses. *Ann. Otol. Rhinol. Laryngol.* 1994 Sep;103(9):699-704.

[74] Michalski JM, Meza J, Breneman JC, et al. Influence of radiation therapy parameters on outcome in children treated with radiation therapy for localized parameningeal rhabdomyosarcoma in Intergroup Rhabdomyosarcoma Study Group trials II through IV. *Int. J. Radiat. Oncol. Biol. Phys.* 2004 Jul 15;59(4):1027-38.

[75] Tefft M, Fernandez C, Donaldson M, Newton W, Moon TE. Incidence of meningeal involvement by rhabdomyosarcoma of the head and neck in children: a report of the Intergroup Rhabdomyosarcoma Study (IRS). *Cancer* 1978 Jul;42(1):253-8.

[76] Wiener ES. Head and neck rhabdomyosarcoma. *Semin. Pediatr. Surg.* 1994 Aug;3(3):203-6.

[77] Hays DM, Lawrence W Jr, Wharam M, et al. Primary reexcision for patients with microscopic residual' tumor following initial excision of sarcomas of trunk and extremity sites. *J. Pediatr. Surg.* 1989 Jan;24(1):5-10.

[78] Cecchetto G, Carli M, Sotti G, et al. Importance of local treatment in pediatric soft tissue sarcomas with microscopic residual after primary surgery: results of the Italian Cooperative Study RMS-88. *Med. Pediatr. Oncol.* 2000 Feb;34(2):97-101.

[79] Thariat J, Italiano A, Peyrade F, et al. Very Late Local Relapse of Ewing's Sarcoma of the Head and Neck treated with Aggressive Multimodal Therapy. *Sarcoma* 2008;2008:854141.

[80] Luu QC, Lasky JL, Moore TB, Nelson S, Wang MB. Treatment of embryonal rhabdomyosarcoma of the sinus and orbit with chemotherapy, radiation, and endoscopic surgery. *J. Pediatr. Surg.* 2006 Jun;41(6):e15-7.

[81] Hays DM, Raney RB, Crist WM, et al. Secondary surgical procedures to evaluate primary tumor status in patients with chemotherapy-responsive stage III and IV sarcomas: a report from the Intergroup Rhabdomyosarcoma Study. *J. Pediatr. Surg.* 1990 Oct;25(10):1100-5.

[82] Godzinski J, Flamant F, Rey A, Praquin MT, Martelli H. Value of postchemotherapy bioptical verification of complete clinical remission in previously incompletely resected (stage I and II pT3) malignant mesenchymal tumors in children: International Society of Pediatric Oncology 1984 Malignant Mesenchymal Tumors Study. *Med. Pediatr. Oncol.* 1994;22(1):22-6.

[83] Sailer SL, Harmon DC, Mankin HJ, Truman JT, Suit HD. Ewing's sarcoma: surgical resection as a prognostic factor. *Int. J. Radiat. Oncol. Biol. Phys.* 1988 Jul;15(1):43-52.

[84] Windfuhr JP. Primitive neuroectodermal tumor of the head and neck: incidence, diagnosis, and management. *Ann. Otol. Rhinol. Laryngol.* 2004 Jul;113(7):533-43.

[85] Allam A, El-Husseiny G, Khafaga Y, et al. Ewing's Sarcoma of the Head and Neck: A Retrospective Analysis of 24 Cases. *Sarcoma* 1999;3(1):11-5.

[86] Sercarz JA, Mark RJ, Nasri S, Wang MB, Tran LM. Pediatric rhabdomyosarcoma of the head and neck. *Int. J. Pediatr. Otorhinolaryngol.* 1995 Jan;31(1):15-22.

[87] Buwalda J, Schouwenburg PF, Blank LE, et al. A novel local treatment strategy for advanced stage head and neck rhabdomyosarcomas in children: results of the AMORE protocol. *Eur. J. Cancer* 2003 Jul;39(11):1594-602.

[88] Raney RB, Anderson JR, Barr FG, et al. Rhabdomyosarcoma and undifferentiated sarcoma in the first two decades of life: a selective review of intergroup rhabdomyosarcoma study group experience and rationale for Intergroup Rhabdomyosarcoma Study V. J Pediatr Hematol Oncol 2001 May;23(4):215-20.

[89] 44. Callender TA, Weber RS, Janjan N, et al. Rhabdomyosarcoma of the nose and paranasal sinuses in adults and children. *Otolaryngol. Head Neck Surg.* 1995 Feb;112(2):252-7.

[90] Newman AN, Rice DH. Rhabdomyosarcoma of the head and neck. *Laryngoscope* 1984 Feb;94(2 Pt 1):234-9.

[91] Arndt CA, Crist WM. Common musculoskeletal tumors of childhood and adolescence. *N. Engl. J. Med.* 1999 Jul 29;341(5):342-52.

[92] Paulino AC, Bauman N, Simon JH, Nguyen TX, Ritchie JM, Tannous R. Local control of parameningeal rhabdomyosarcoma: outcomes in non-complete responders to chemoradiation. *Med. Pediatr. Oncol.* 2003 Aug;41(2):118-22.

[93] Buwalda J, Blank LE, Schouwenburg PF, et al. The AMORE protocol as salvage treatment for non-orbital head and neck rhabdomyosarcoma in children. *Eur. J. Surg. Oncol.* 2004 Oct;30(8):884-92.

[94] McTiernan AM, Cassoni AM, Driver D, Michelagnoli MP, Kilby AM, Whelan JS. Improving Outcomes After Relapse in Ewing's Sarcoma: Analysis of 114 Patients From a Single Institution. *Sarcoma* 2006;2006:83548.

[95] Temeck BK, Wexler LH, Steinberg SM, McClure LL, Horowitz M, Pass HI. Metastasectomy for sarcomatous pediatric histologies: results and prognostic factors. *Ann. Thorac. Surg.* 1995 Jun;59(6):1385-9; discussion 1390.

In: Sarcoma
Editor: Eric J. Butler

ISBN: 978-1-62100-362-5
© 2012 Nova Science Publishers, Inc.

Chapter VIII

Gastrointestinal Kaposi's Sarcoma: Diagnosis and Clinical Features

Naoyoshi Nagata[1], Ryo Nakashima[1], Sou Nishimura[2], Naoki Asayma[1], Kazuhiro Watanabe[1], Koh Imbe[1], Tomoyuki Yada[2], Junichi Akiyama[1], Hirohisa Yazaki[2], Shinichi Oka[2] and Naomi Uemura[2]

[1]Department of Gastroenterology and Hepatology, Division of AIDS Clinical Center (ACC), National Center for Global Health and Medicine, Tokyo, 162-8655, Japan
[2]Department of Gastroenterology and Hepatology, National Center for Global Health and Medicine, Kohnodai Hospital, Chiba, 272-0827, Japan

Abstract

BACKGROUND: Kaposi's sarcoma (KS) is a rare malignant tumor, but often occurs in patients with AIDS. The gastrointestinal (GI) tract is the third most commonly affected site after the skin and the lymph nodes. Early diagnosis of GI-KS is important because advanced GI lesions may cause hemorrhage, perforation, and obstruction. However, the clinical characteristics of GI-KS have not been fully studied. The aim of this study was to clarify the key clinical factors for the diagnosis of GI-KS.

METHODS: We retrospectively reviewed the cases of 311 HIV-infected patients who had undergone endoscopy between 2003 and 2007. Endoscopic images of tissue biopsies and supplementary immunological staining were used in the diagnosis of GI-KS. Clinical parameters such as HIV infection route, fecal occult blood test (FOBT) results, GI symptoms, CD4 lymphocyte count, and the viral load of KS-associated herpes virus (KSHV) in the blood were assessed. Skin lesions and extracutaneous spread of KS were examined prior to endoscopy.

RESULTS: Twenty-seven of the 311 patients had a diagnosis of GI-KS. Endoscopic biopsy was performed on a total of 238 lesions suspected to be GI-KS, of these, 162 lesions (68.1%) were confirmed to be GI-KS. Common organ involvement in the GI-KS patients was the stomach (11 patients), duodenum (10), colon (7), esophagus (4), rectum (3), and terminal ileum (2). Age and sex were not significant factors but CD4 count was significantly lower in patients with GI-KS than those without GI-KS (median KS+ 69 vs. KS- 270.5, $p<0.01$).

Among 27 patients with GI-KS, men who have sex with men (MSM) was the most frequent HIV infection route in patients with GI-KS (21/27). FOBT was positive in 17% of cases involving the upper GI tract and in 30% of those involving the lower intestinal tract. GI symptoms were observed in 19%. KSHV viral loads were positive in 50%, and the median level was 900 copy/ml. Other organs involvement of KS were the skin (23), lymph nodes (15), oral cavity (4), respiratory tract (3), conjunctiva (2), and liver (1). In 4 patients, all asymptomatic MSM patients, KS lesions were found only in the GI tract.

CONCLUSION: Upper endoscopy should be considered for patients especially with particularly low CD4 counts who are MSM even when patients are asymptomatic or FOBT results are negative. Several biopsies with immunohistochemical staining are recommended for pathological confirmation. This strategy can lead to early diagnosis and treatment of GI-KS.

Introduction

Kaposi sarcoma was first reported by the dermatologist Dr. Moritz Kaposi in 1872 [1] and was described as idiopathic multiple pigmented sarcoma of the skin before being named Kaposi's sarcoma (KS). KS was initially considered to be a rare malignant tumor that develops in the elderly in the Mediterranean region. However, since the 1980s, KS has been frequently observed among patients with human immunodeficiency virus (HIV), especially among men who have sex with men (MSM) [2, 3]. Currently, 4 types of KS are recognized: classic type- seen among the Mediterranean elderly, rapidly progressive endemic or African-type affecting children in Africa, immunosuppression-associated type in individuals with a previous organ transplant or a history of immunosuppressant therapy, and acquired immunodeficiency syndrome (AIDS)-associated type [4–8].

Human herpes virus 8 (HHV-8) was newly discovered from a KS lesion in 1994, and is thought to be the pathogenesis of KS [9]. Because the majority of KS patients are homosexuals, and not heterosexuals or females, and because the HHV-8 gene is isolated from semen and saliva, the route of infection appears to be sexual contact [8]. The frequency of KS occurrence in HIV patients is 20,000 times higher than in uninfected individuals, 300 times higher than individuals with other immunodeficiency disorders, and approximately 20–30 times higher among homosexual or bisexual men with AIDS compared to heterosexual individuals with AIDS [8]. Although the incidence of KS in American men with AIDS decreased from 40% in 1981 to less than 20%in 1992,[10] it remains the most common AIDS-associated malignancy.

The gastrointestinal (GI) tract is the third most commonly affected site after the skin and the lymph nodes in KS [11-15]. Early diagnosis of GI-KS is important because advanced GI lesions may cause hemorrhage, perforation, and obstruction requiring emergent treatment [13,16–18]. However, a limited number of studies have reported on GI-KS and the clinical features of the disease have not been fully clarified [13–16, 19]. Moreover, although endoscopic examination is clearly a valuable diagnostic method for GI-KS, its indications remain to be determined. The aim of this study, therefore, was to clarify the key clinical factors for early diagnosis of GI-KS in HIV-infected patients.

Methods

Patient Selection

We retrospectively reviewed the cases of 311 HIV-infected patients who had undergone endoscopy between 2003 and 2007 at the National Center for Global Health and Medicine (NCGM), a 900-bed hospital located in the Tokyo metropolitan area and the largest referral center for HIV/AIDS in Japan.

Written informed consent was obtained from all patients prior to performing endoscopy and biopsy.

Diagnosis of KS

Gastrointestinal Tract

We performed biopsy when abnormal findings were encountered on endoscopy. GI-KS was suspected based on endoscopic appearance, such as the presence of submucosal nodules, polypoid nodules, or a deep red mucosa (Figure 1a–f), as previously reported [19–21]. GI-KS was defined as the presence of proliferating spindle cells in the biopsy specimens on hematoxylin and eosin (HE) staining (Figure 2a). The spindle cells were consistently positive on immunohistochemical staining for D2-40 (Figure 2b), CD34 (Figure 2c), and human herpes virus 8 (HHV8) (Figure 2d), as previously reported [22,23]. To clarify the common involvement of the GI tract, we assessed the presence of lesions including in the esophagus, stomach, duodenum, terminal ileum, colon and rectum.

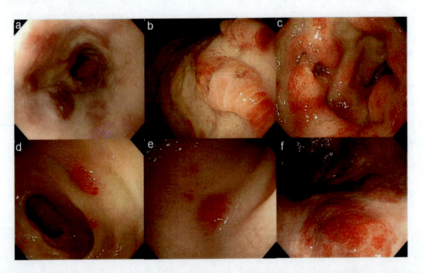

Figure 1. Endoscopic appearance of gastrointestinal Kaposi's sarcoma (KS), lesions of which can develop anywhere in the GI tract. (a) Multiple dark reddish flat mucosa in the esophagus. (b) Submusosal nodules with erosion in the stomach. (c) Submucosal nodules with circumferential ulcer in the duodenum. Strong reddish polypoid nodule in (d) the ileum and (f) the sigmoid colon. (f) Submucosal nodule in the rectum.

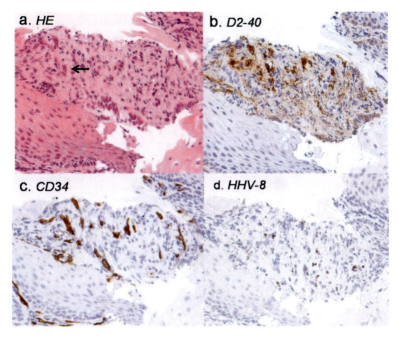

Figure 2. Pathological features of GI-KS. (a) Spindle-cell proliferation found in the submucosa on hematoxylin and eosin (HE) staining. (b, c) Immunohistochemical staining reveals strong co-expression of CD34 and D2-40. The vascular gaps are lined with endothelial cells on staining for CD34 and D2-40. (d) Some endothelial cells are positive for human herpes virus 8 (HHV8).

Cutaneous and Extracutaneous Involvement

Before endoscopy, we examined patients for cutaneous involvement. Patients found to have skin lesions were further examined for the presence of lesions in the oral cavity and conjunctiva. Abdominal and chest computed tomography (CT) was used to determine extracutaneous involvement. Positron emission tomography (PET) was performed for the lesions that were difficult to evaluate with CT.

Clinical Parameters

HIV infection routes were determined by the medical staff who questioned each patient on the first visit to our hospital. Routes were classified into six categories: homosexual; bisexual; heterosexual; drug user; hemophiliac; and unknown. We defined sexual behavior as MSM or heterosexual. Patients who were not homosexual or bisexual were regarded as heterosexual.

A fecal occult blood test (FOBT) was conducted before endoscopy. Gastrointestinal symptoms were recorded by the doctor who interviewed each patient prior to endoscopy. Individuals whose notes contained no such record were regarded as symptom free. $CD4^+$ cell counts within 1 week of endoscopy were reviewed, and the viral load of Kaposi's Sarcoma-Associated Herpes virus (KSHV) in the blood as determined by real-time quantitative PCR as previously reported [24] was examined. The minimum detection level was 200 copies/mL of plasma. A positive result for real-time KSHV PCR was defined as ≥200 copies/mL.

Results

Baseline Characteristics

Twenty-seven (8.7%) of the 311 patients were diagnosed with GI-KS. Of the 311 patients, no significant differences were noted in age and sex between two groups (Median age, GI-KS+ 41 vs GI-KS- 42, p=0.71) (male/ female, GI-KS+ 262/ 22 vs 27/0, p=0.13). CD4 count was significantly lower in patients with GI-KS than those without GI-KS (median GI-KS+ 69 vs. GI-KS- 270.5, p<0.01).

Clinical Characteristics of Gastrointestinal Kaposi's Sarcoma

Endoscopic biopsy was performed on a total of 238 lesions suspected to be KS, among which 162 lesions (68.1%) were confirmed to be KS. GI lesions were found in the stomach (11 patients), duodenum (10), colon (7), esophagus (4), rectum (3), and terminal ileum (2).

Characteristics of the 27 GI-KS patients are shown in Table 1. The most frequent route of HIV infection was MSM. FOBT was positive in the upper GI tract in 7.6% of cases and in the lower GI tract in 23.6% of cases. GI symptoms were noted in 19% (5/27) of the GI-KS patients as follows: diarrhea (2), lower abdominal pain (2), and epigastric pain (1). KSHV-PCR results were positive in 50% of the patients, and the median level was 900 (range, 300–70,000) copy/ml.

Table 1. Clinical characteristics of GI-KS patients (N = 27)

Age- Median (IQR)	41 (34, 55)
Sex (Male)- No.	27
MSM- No.	21
Positive FOBT- No. (%).	
Upper GI tract- No. (%)	1/13 (7.6)
Lower GI tract- No. (%)	5/22 (23.6)
KS organ distribution	
Skin- No. (%)	23 (85)
Lymph nodes- No. (%)	15 (56)
Others*- No. (%)	7 (26)
Respiratory tract- No. (%)	3 (11)
With GI symptoms- No.	5
CD4 lymphocyte count- Median (IQR)	69 (16, 176)
KSHV PCR positive- No. (%)	10/20 (50)

Abbreviations: IQR: Inter-quartile range, MSM: men who have sex with men, FOBT: Fecal occult blood test, GI: Gastrointestinal, KSHV: Kaposi's sarcoma-associated herpes virus, Others* include oral cavity 4 (15%), conjuctiva 2 (7%), and liver 2 (7%).

Table 2. GI-KS patients without any other organs involvement

	Case 1	Case 2	Case 3	Case 4
KS-GI involvement	Stomach	Stomach and duodenum	Duodenum	Stomach
Age- years	46	34	32	46
Sex	male	male	male	male
HIV infection route	homosexual	bisexual	homosexual	bisexual
GI symptoms	None	None	None	None
CD4 (cells/µl)	250	10	11	15
KSHV (copy/ml)	<200	<200	<200	<200

Organ involvement in the 27 GI-KS patients was highest in the skin, followed in order by the lymph nodes, oral cavity, respiratory tract, conjunctiva, and liver (Table 1). There were 4 GI-KS patients without any other organs involvement (Table 2). They were all MSM patients. These patients were asymptomatic at the time of diagnosis and opted to undergo endoscopy during annual check-ups. Their KSHV-PCR levels were all within the normal range.

Discussion

Although the rate of KS has fallen dramatically since the advent of highly active antiretroviral therapy (HAART) [25,26], KS remains the most common malignancy in patients with HIV infection [27]. In this study, we performed endoscopic observation of 311 HIV-infected patients, 27 (8.7%) of whom were diagnosed with GI-KS. Endoscopy is extremely useful for the early diagnosis of GI-KS because it enables minimal mucosal changes to be detected as well as biopsies to be taken. It also minimizes the advancement and avoidesthe onset of emergent symptoms such as hemorrhage, perforation, and obstruction [13,16-18]. However, endoscopy is not recommended for all patients because of considerations of cost and invasiveness. This raises the question, which patients should be examined by endoscopy? What are other key clinical features, besides endoscopic observation, that can be used to diagnose GI-KS? What are the crucial points to remember during endoscopic observation? The present study sought to answer these questions.

The comparison of patients with and without GI-KS showed no significant differences by age or sex. On the other hand, the median value of CD4 in GI-KS patients was 69 (range, 7–347) and thus significantly lower than that of patients without GI-KS at 270.5. Interestingly, a recent report indicated that, in the era of HAART, CD4 levels in KS patients are relatively high [28,29]; however, the relationship between GI-KS and CD 4 levels has not been fully investigated. It is necessary to pay extra attention to GI lesions during endoscopic observation of patients with cutaneous KS and a low CD 4 level.

We hypothesized that, besides endoscopic observation, FOBT and blood KSHV-PCR results would be useful for the diagnosis of GI-KS. FOBT is a simple test that has been performed widely to detect malignant disease; however, the results here showed a fairly low rate (25%). Even though some studies suggest that quantitative KSHV assay is useful for monitoring KS evolution [24,30], negative KSHV results were obtained in half of our cases. In addition, 80% of the GI-KS patients were asymptomatic, which accords with the findings of previous reports [19–21]. For these reasons, it is difficult to predict GI-KS on the basis of FOBT and KSHV results and presence of GI symptoms. MSM with AIDS are reported to have an approximately 20–30 times greater risk of developing KS [8], and we found that 80% of our GI-KS patients were MSM. However, we only investigated clinical factors of GI-KS cases, and therefore, it is recommended that case-control studies be conducted to reveal clinical findings predictive of GI-KS.

It remains unclear whether an upper or lower GI endoscopy is an appropriate procedure to search for GI-KS. Because stomach and duodenum involvement was a common finding in the present study, an upper GI endoscopy does appear to be the first option to consider. This view is supported by previous studies reporting a high prevalence of KS in the upper GI tract (31).

Previous studies reported that only 19–31% of endoscopically biopsied lesions tested positive for KS [19,32-34]. The submucosal appearance of KS is considered to account for this poor diagnostic yield from standard forcep biopsies [32–34]. However, in the present study, we could achieve a high diagnostic rate of approximately 70% by combining biopsies from a number of sites and immunohistochemical staining for D2-40, CD34, and HHV8. In addition, no biopsy-related complications such as bleeding and perforation were observed, indicating that biopsy is a safe diagnostic procedure for GI-KS. We recommend that more than one biopsy be taken from GI lesions suspected to be GI-KS and that pathological information and immunohistochemical staining be obtained from a pathologist.

AIDS-related KS can occur in the GI tract in the absence of cutaneous disease [35]. In the present study, 4 of the 27 GI-KS patients showed no cutaneous and extracutaneous involvement. Furthermore, these 4 patients were all MSM with no GI symptoms. This indicates that these cases would not have been detected if endoscopy had not been performed. The relationship between KS skin lesions and extracutaneous lesions and their etiology remain to be fully clarified.

Conclusion

To diagnose GI-KS at an early stage, clinical factors need to be considered before endoscopy. Patients with low CD4 counts and MSM patients are advisable to perform endoscopy even with a negative FOBT or asymptomatic. Upper GI tract is recommended for indication for endoscopy to detect GI-KS and biopsy should be taken from lesions. To evaluate biopsy specimens, immunohistochemical staining needs to be carried out. These diagnostic strategies could help to make the early diagnosis and treatment of GI-KS possible.

Acknowledgments

We wish to express our gratitude to Hisae Kawashiro (clinical research coordinator) for help with collecting data in this study.

Funding
This work was supported by Sachi foundation.

References

[1] Braun M. Classics in Oncology. Idiopathic multiple pigmented sarcoma of the skin by Kaposi. *CA Cancer J. Clin.* 1982;32(6):340-7.
[2] Friedman-Kien AE, Laubenstein LJ, Rubinstein P, Buimovici-Klein E, Marmor M, Stahl R, Spigland I, Kim KS, Zolla-Pazner S. Disseminated Kaposi's sarcoma in homosexual men. *Ann. Intern. Med.* 1982;96(6 Pt 1):693-700.
[3] Friedman-Kien AE, Laubenstein L, Marmor M, et al. Kaposi's sarcoma and pneumocystis pneumonia among homosexual men: New York City and California. *MMWR Morb. Mortal Wkly. Rep.* 1981;30:305-8.
[4] Antman K, Chang Y. Kaposi's sarcoma. *N. Engl. J. Med.* 2000; 342(14):1027-38.
[5] DiGiovanna JJ, Safai B. Kaposi's sarcoma: retrospective study of 90 cases with particular emphasis on the familial occurrences, ethnic background and prevalence of other diseases. *Am. J. Med.* 1981;71:779-83.
[6] Montagnino G, Bencini PL, Tarantino A, Caputo R, Ponticelli C. Clinical features and course of Kaposi's sarcoma in kidney transplant patients: report of 13 cases. *Am. J. Nephrol.* 1994;14(2):121-6.
[7] Lesnoni La Parola I, Masini C, Nanni G, Diociaiuti A, Panocchia N, Cerimele D. Kaposi's sarcoma in renal-transplant recipients: experience at the Catholic University in Rome, 1988-1996. *Dermatology.* 1997;194(3):229-33.
[8] Beral V, Peterman TA, Berkelman RL, Jaffe HW. Kaposi's sarcoma among persons with AIDS: a sexually transmitted infection? *Lancet.* 1990;335(8682):123-8.

[9] Chang Y, Cesarman E, Pessin MS, Lee F, Culpepper J, Knowles DM, Moore PS. Identification of herpes virus-like DNA sequences in AIDS-associated Kaposi's sarcoma. *Science.* 1994;266(5192):1865-9.
[10] Biggar RJ, Rabkin CS. The epidemiology of AIDS--related neoplasms. *Hematol. Oncol. Clin. North Am.* 1996;10(5):997-1010.
[11] Dezube BJ. Clinical presentation and natural history of AIDS-related Kaposi's sarcoma. *Hematol. Oncol. Clin. North Am.* 1996;10(5):1023-9.
[12] Ngendahayo P, Mets T, Bugingo G, Parkin DM. Kaposi's sarcoma in Rwanda: clinico-pathological and epidemiological aspects. *Bull. Cancer.* 1989;76(4):383-94.
[13] Danzig B, Brandt LJ, Reinus JF, Klein RS. Gastrointestinal malignancy in patients with AIDS. *Am. J. Gastroenterol.* 1991;86(6):715-8.
[14] Laine L, Amerian J, Rarick M, Harb M, Gill PS. The response of symptomatic gastrointestinal Kaposi's sarcoma to chemotherapy: a prospective evaluation using an endoscopic method of disease quantification. *Am. J. Gastroenterol.* 1990;85(8):959-61.
[15] Ioachim HL, Adsay V, Giancotti FR, Dorsett B, Melamed J. Kaposi's sarcoma of internal organs. A multi-parameter study of 86 cases. *Cancer.* 1995;75(6):1376-85.
[16] Chor PJ, Santa Cruz DJ. Kaposi's sarcoma. A clinicopathologic review and differential diagnosis. *J. Cutan. Pathol.* 1992 Feb;19(1):6-20.
[17] Yoshida EM, Chan NH, Chan-Yan C, Baird RM. Perforation of the jejunum secondary to AIDS-related gastrointestinal Kaposi's sarcoma. *Can. J. Gastroenterol.* 1997 Jan-Feb;11(1):38-40.
[18] Nagata N, Yazaki H, Oka S. Kaposi's Sarcoma Presenting as a Bulky Tumor Mass of the Colon. *Clin. Gastroenterol. Hepatol.* 2011;9(5):A22.
[19] Friedman SL, Wright TL, Altman DF. Gastrointestinal Kaposi's sarcoma in patients with acquired immunodeficiency syndrome. Endoscopic and autopsy findings. *Gastroenterology.* 1985;89(1):102-8.
[20] Ahmed N, Nelson RS, Goldstein HM, Sinkovics JG. Kaposi's sarcoma of the stomach and duodenum: endoscopic and roentgenologic correlations. *Gastrointest. Endosc.* 1975;21(4):149-152.
[21] Weprin L, Zollinger R, Clausen K, Thomas FB. Kaposi's sarcoma: endoscopic observations of gastric and colon involvement. *J. Clin. Gastroenterol.* 1982;4(4):357-60..
[22] Kahn HJ, Bailey D, Marks A. Monoclonal antibody D2-40, a new marker of lymphatic endothelium, reacts with Kaposi's sarcoma and a subset of angiosarcomas. *Mod. Pathol.* 2002;15(4):434-40.

[23] Kaiserling E. Immunohistochemical identification of lymph vessels with D2-40 in diagnostic pathology. *Pathologe.* 2004;25(5):362-74.
[24] Whitby D, Howard MR, Tenant-Flowers M, Brink NS, Copas A, Boshoff C, Hatzioannou T, Suggett FE, Aldam DM, Denton AS, et al. Detection of Kaposi sarcoma associated herpes virus in peripheral blood of HIV-infected individuals and progression to Kaposi's sarcoma. *Lancet.* 1995;346(8978):799-802.
[25] Buchacz K, Baker RK, Palella FJ Jr, Chmiel JS, Lichtenstein KA, Novak RM, Wood KC, Brooks JT; HOPS Investigators. AIDS-defining opportunistic illnesses in US patients, 1994-2007: a cohort study. *AIDS.* 2010;24:1549-1559.
[26] Engels EA, Pfeiffer RM, Goedert JJ, Virgo P, McNeel TS, Scoppa SM, Biggar RJ; for the HIV/AIDS Cancer Match Study. Trends in cancer risk among people with AIDS in the United States, 1980-2002. *AIDS.* 2006;20:1645-1654.
[27] Mocroft A, Kirk O, Clumeck N, Gargalianos-Kakolyris P, Trocha H, Chentsova N, Antunes F, Stellbrink HJ, Phillips AN, Lundgren JD. The changing pattern of Kaposi sarcoma in patients with HIV, 1994-2003: the EuroSIDA Study. *Cancer.* 2004;100(12):2644-54.
[28] Crum-Cianflone NF, Hullsiek KH, Ganesan A, Weintrob A, Okulicz JF, Agan BK; Infectious Disease Clinical Research Program HIV Working Group. Is Kaposi's sarcoma occurring at higher CD4 cell counts over the course of the HIV epidemic? *AIDS.* 2010;24(18):2881-3.
[29] Lodi S, Guiguet M, Costagliola D, Fisher M, de Luca A, Porter K; CASCADE Collaboration. Kaposi sarcoma incidence and survival among HIV-infected homosexual men after HIV seroconversion. *J. Natl. Cancer Inst.* 2010;102(11):784-92. Epub 2010 May 4.
[30] Moore PS, Kingsley LA, Holmberg SD, Spira T, Gupta P, Hoover DR, Parry JP, Conley LJ, Jaffe HW, Chang Y. Kaposi's sarcoma-associated herpes virus infection prior to onset of Kaposi's sarcoma. *AIDS.* 1996;10(2):175-80.
[31] Saltz RK, Kurtz RC, Lightdale CJ, Myskowski P, Cunningham-Rundles S, Urmacher C, Safai B. Kaposi's sarcoma. Gastrointestinal involvement correlation with skin findings and immunologic function. *Dig. Dis. Sci.* 1984;29:817–23.
[32] Boyd GD, Shabot JM, Pollard RB, Gourley WK. Endoscopic evolution of gastric Kaposi's sarcoma. *Gastrointest. Endosc.* 1987;33(6):450-3.

[33] Cosnes J, Darmoni SJ, Evard D, Le Quintrec Y. Value of digestive endoscopic examination in acquired immunodeficiency syndrome (45 cases). *Ann. Gastroenterol. Hepatol.* (Paris). 1986;22(3):123-8.
[34] Kolios G, Kaloterakis A, Filiotou A, Nakos A, Hadziyannis S. Gastroscopic findings in Mediterranean Kaposi's sarcoma (non-AIDS). *Gastrointest. Endosc.* 1994;42:336–9.

Index

A

acid, 10, 22, 77, 81, 102, 127, 128
acidic, 125, 126, 127, 128
acidity, 126, 128, 136
acquired immunodeficiency syndrome, 30, 155, 163, 165
acute leukemia, 22
adamantinoma, 18, 24
adhesion, 70, 92
adipose tissue, 125, 126
adolescents, 10, 17, 18, 101, 109, 148
adulthood, 18, 21
adults, xii, 8, 18, 24, 32, 33, 34, 37, 40, 41, 139, 151
Africa, 37, 39, 155
aggressive behavior, 39
aggressiveness, xii, 24, 140
AIDS, xiii, 36, 37, 38, 40, 41, 44, 45, 46, 49, 51, 53, 54, 55, 56, 58, 59, 60, 62, 153, 155, 160, 161, 162, 163, 164, 165
airways, 42
alanine, 77, 78
alters, 104
amino, ix, 64, 66, 76, 77, 78, 80, 82
amino acid, ix, 64, 66, 76, 77, 78, 80, 82
amputation, xi, 27, 34, 108, 109, 115, 118, 133
analgesic, 112

anatomic site, 26, 109
anatomy, 94
angiofibroma, 3, 4
angiogenesis, 91, 94, 104, 111
angiosarcoma, 12, 18, 39, 58
anhydrase, 128
antibiotic, 69
antibody, 61, 106, 163
anti-cancer, 102, 111, 132
anti-inflammatory drugs, 56
antitumor, ix, x, xi, 63, 64, 65, 66, 68, 69, 71, 74, 76, 77, 78, 79, 80, 81, 103, 108, 111, 112, 125
antitumor agent, ix, x, 63, 64, 65, 66, 69, 74, 80
aphonia, 43
apoptosis, 37, 91, 105, 106, 127, 128
appendicitis, 42
appendicular skeleton, x, 108, 109
Argentina, 107, 112, 120
arteries, 27
arthrodesis, 34
arthroplasty, 27, 34
ascites, 134
aspartate, 82
aspiration, 12, 141, 145, 149
assessment, 24, 93, 102, 142
asymptomatic, xiv, 41, 42, 45, 46, 154, 159, 160, 161
ataxia, 48

Index

ATP, 75, 83
autopsy, 45, 163
axial skeleton, 44

B

bacillus, 47
back pain, 43
bacteria, 125, 132
base, 99, 100, 102, 134, 143, 147
basement membrane, 96, 105
basic research, x, 86, 90, 93, 95, 122, 125, 133
behaviors, x, 86, 87, 92, 94, 96
beneficial effect, 66
benefits, xiii, 140
benign, vii, viii, 2, 3, 6, 8, 10, 11, 18, 19, 21, 23, 24, 62, 99, 126
benign tumors, vii, 2, 18, 126
bile, 78
biocompatibility, 96
biological activities, 125
biological activity, 11, 105
biological behavior, 94
biomaterials, x, 86, 96
biopsy, viii, xiii, 2, 12, 14, 17, 25, 32, 48, 50, 57, 115, 116, 132, 141, 145, 147, 149, 154, 156, 158, 161
biosynthesis, x, 64, 76
bleeding, viii, 36, 44, 161
blood, vii, xiii, 1, 7, 19, 34, 50, 51, 52, 69, 74, 78, 90, 154, 158, 160
blood pressure, 78
blood vessels, vii, 1, 7, 50, 51, 52, 69, 90
blood-brain barrier, 74
body weight, 69, 70
bone, vii, viii, x, xii, 1, 2, 8, 9, 11, 14, 15, 17, 18, 19, 20, 21, 22, 23, 24, 25, 26, 27, 29, 31, 32, 34, 41, 44, 45, 47, 60, 86, 88, 93, 94, 98, 99, 101, 103, 105, 108, 109, 117, 118, 124, 126, 130, 131, 132, 133, 139
bone cancer, x, 18, 26, 86, 108, 109
bone form, 20, 24
bone marrow, 22, 44

bone scan, 14
bone tumors, 20, 23, 25, 27, 109, 131, 133
bones, xi, 10, 17, 21, 22, 24, 44, 47, 88, 99, 124, 142, 148
bowel, 41
brain, 18, 42, 56, 74, 76, 82, 83
branching, 9
breast cancer, 6, 18, 81

C

calcification, 19, 21, 24
calcifications, 9, 11
calcium, 78
CAM, 52
cancer, x, xi, 6, 17, 26, 29, 37, 38, 48, 64, 65, 68, 76, 80, 81, 86, 87, 88, 89, 90, 92, 93, 94, 95, 96, 97, 98, 102, 103, 104, 105, 107, 108, 109, 121, 122, 127, 128, 132, 133, 135, 136, 164
cancer cells, 90, 92, 96, 97, 102, 127, 128
candidates, 96
capillary, 4, 8
carbon, 89, 100
carboxyl, 51
carcinogen, 132
carcinogenesis, 132, 136
carcinogenicity, 132
carcinoma, 22, 44
cardiac muscle, 78
carnosine, 83
cartilage, vii, 1, 19, 21, 86, 93, 94, 98, 99, 103, 104
cartilaginous, 21, 24
Caucasians, 18
cavernous hemangiomas, 47
CDC, 37
cell biology, 92
cell culture, 101
cell death, 127, 136
cell differentiation, 4, 83
cell invasion, 104
cell line, 66, 83, 92, 93, 102, 103, 106, 111, 122, 134

Index

cell lines, 66, 83, 92, 93, 102, 103, 106, 111, 122
cell membranes, 80
central nervous system (CNS), 42, 143
cerebellum, 42, 73
cerebrum, 42
cervical cancer, 132
challenges, x, 86, 88, 91, 92
chemical, 6, 74, 78, 87
chemicals, 136
chemoprevention, 103
chemotherapeutic agent, 69, 76
chemotherapeutics, 55
chemotherapy, vii, viii, ix, x, xi, xii, xiii, 2, 9, 10, 11, 13, 15, 16, 17, 19, 21, 22, 23, 26, 27, 28, 29, 33, 34, 55, 56, 63, 64, 65, 66, 68, 76, 80, 81, 86, 88, 89, 97, 100, 105, 108, 109, 110, 112, 115, 117, 120, 140, 141, 143, 144, 146, 147, 150, 151, 163
chest radiography, 117
children, vii, xii, 5, 7, 9, 10, 17, 18, 24, 27, 33, 37, 39, 40, 41, 56, 101, 124, 132, 133, 139, 143, 147, 148, 149, 150, 151, 152, 155
Chile, 57
China, 58, 85
chondroblastoma, 21, 24
chondrocyte, 91
chondroma, 4, 20, 21
chondrosarcoma, vii, x, 1, 4, 86, 87, 88, 89, 90, 91, 92, 93, 94, 95, 96, 97, 98, 99, 100, 101, 102, 103, 104, 105, 106, 127, 136
chromosome, 6, 10, 18
chronic lymphocytic leukemia, 39, 47
chylothorax, 44
classification, 3, 7, 12, 19, 20, 21, 99, 131
claudication, 116
clinical application, 90, 110, 122, 125, 128, 129
clinical examination, 14
clinical presentation, 22, 41, 49, 86, 87, 88, 92, 97, 108
clinical symptoms, 43, 56

clinical syndrome, ix, 36
closure, 129
clusters, 51
coagulopathy, 47
coal tar, 125
collaboration, 97
collagen, 93
colon, xiv, 154, 156, 158, 163
colonization, 94
comparative analysis, 133
complete blood count, 119
complexity, 96
complications, 15, 88, 108, 161
compounds, 134
compression, 7, 16, 44, 59
computed tomography, viii, 2, 11, 143, 147, 157
conjunctiva, xiv, 44, 154, 157, 159
connective tissue, 2
contamination, 25
control group, 69, 71, 129
control measures, 144
correlation, 21, 34, 59, 101, 164
correlations, 121, 163
cortex, viii, 2, 22, 24, 115
cosmetic, xiii, 140, 142
cough, 41, 43
cranial nerve, 142
cryosurgery, 88, 99
CSF, 110, 119
CT scan, 17, 44, 48
Cuba, 35
culture, x, 86, 92, 93, 96, 102, 105, 125
cure, xii, 22, 26, 140, 143, 144, 148
cycles, 144
cyclophosphamide, 28, 29
cyst, 20, 21
cytogenetics, 12
cytokines, 41, 111, 121
cytology, 12
cytomegalovirus, 46
cytometry, 12, 31, 32
cytoplasm, 125
cytotoxicity, 111

D

database, 32
death rate, 87, 88
debulking surgery, 142, 149
deep venous thrombosis, 15
defects, 27
deficiency, 6, 60, 62
demonstrations, 56
deposits, 44
depth, 5, 10
derivatives, x, 64, 71, 78, 81, 96
dermatologist, 36, 154
dermatome, 45, 60
dermis, 50
destruction, 19, 24, 50, 94
detectable, xi, 10, 108, 109
detection, viii, 2, 12, 25, 32, 45, 62, 135, 158
detoxification, 76
diaphysis, 22, 116
diarrhea, 41, 54, 158
differential diagnosis, viii, 24, 36, 47, 51, 163
diffusion, 27, 79, 94
dioxin, 6
disability, xi, 124
discomfort, 43
disease model, 96
disease progression, 110
diseases, xii, 5, 47, 109, 140, 162
disintegrin, 106
disorder, 47
disseminated intravascular coagulation, 61
distribution, xii, 49, 82, 89, 92, 103, 139, 159
DNA, 12, 30, 31, 32, 37, 58, 110, 111, 112, 113, 119, 121, 125, 163
DNA ploidy, 12, 31, 32
DNAs, 112
docetaxel, 16, 29
doctors, 46, 49, 57
dogs, x, 107, 108, 109, 110, 112, 119, 121
dopamine, 83
drainage, 13
drug delivery, ix, 64
drug efflux, 66, 76
drug resistance, 66, 67, 91, 94, 95, 102, 105
drug testing, 102
drugs, xii, 16, 19, 65, 71, 73, 76, 84, 92, 102, 140
duodenum, xiv, 41, 154, 156, 158, 159, 161, 163
dura mater, 42
dysphagia, 43
dysplasia, 20

E

Eastern Europe, 37, 38
E-cadherin, 95, 105
ECM, 92, 94, 96, 102
edema, 43, 44, 54
effusion, 37, 42, 44
electron, 12
emboli, 146
embolization, 146
emission, viii, 2, 32, 157
emotional distress, 42
enchondroma, 21
encoding, 110, 121
endoscopy, xiii, xiv, 154, 155, 156, 157, 158, 159, 160, 161
endothelial cells, 37, 50, 51, 157
endothelium, 51, 61, 163
energy, 89, 128, 135
engineering, x, 86, 91, 95, 97, 105
England, 98, 103
environment, xi, 96, 108
environmental factors, 95
enzymes, 74, 83, 128
epicardium, 45
epidemic, 36, 41, 57, 59, 62, 164
epidemiology, 30, 109, 163
epiphysis, 24
epithelial ovarian cancer, 102
epithelium, 92, 95
Epstein Barr, 7
erosion, 24, 156
erythrocyte sedimentation rate, 23

esophagus, xiv, 41, 154, 156, 158
ethical issues, 112
ethnic background, 162
etiology, vii, 1, 6, 17, 161
evidence, 5, 9, 10, 11, 13, 14, 21, 25, 32, 42, 71, 89, 92, 94, 95, 113, 115, 116, 117, 118, 120, 132, 146
evolution, 160, 164
examinations, 48
excision, viii, xi, xiii, 2, 9, 12, 14, 15, 27, 55, 88, 108, 119, 125, 128, 140, 143, 146, 150
excitation, 125, 126, 129, 135
exclusion, 9
excretion, 78
exposure, 6, 8, 47, 126, 127
extracellular matrix, 92, 94, 98
extracts, 110
extrusion, 128

F

families, 130
family members, 75
fat, vii, 1, 8, 11, 46
FDA, 55, 132
FDA approval, 132
female rat, 19, 37
femur, 19, 21, 34, 44
fertility, 28
fever, 23, 41, 54, 119
fibroblasts, 19, 34
fibrosarcoma, 3, 5, 7, 9, 11, 18, 21, 31
fibrous dysplasia, 18
fibula, 24, 44, 124
fish, 77
fluid, 126, 127, 128
fluorescence, 125, 126, 128, 129, 137
food, x, 64, 65, 80
formation, 7, 21, 96, 102, 127, 128, 136
fractures, 17, 27, 44
fragments, 113
France, 102
functional analysis, 82
fusion, 26

G

gamma globulin, 61
gastrointestinal bleeding, 41
gastrointestinal involvement, 39, 41
gastrointestinal tract, viii, 30, 36, 37, 40, 49
gel, 55
gene expression, 37, 104, 109
gene therapy, vii, xi, 108, 110, 111, 114, 116, 117, 118, 120, 121, 122
gene transfer, 111
genes, 52, 106, 115, 117, 118, 119, 120
genetic alteration, 6
genetics, 92, 99, 101
gland, 9, 45
glial cells, 83
glioma, 73, 82
glucose, 37
glutamate, x, 64, 71, 72, 73, 74, 76, 81, 82, 83, 84
glutamine, 82
glutathione, ix, 64, 74, 75, 80, 83
glycogen, 21
glycolysis, 127, 128, 136
grades, 93
grading, 12, 13, 98
granules, 125
granulomas, 47
gravity, 87
Greece, 58
growth, 24, 34, 37, 39, 42, 69, 81, 95, 102, 103, 104, 109, 111
growth arrest, 34
growth rate, 37
guidance, 25
guidelines, 10, 14, 30, 31

H

HAART, 46, 55, 56, 57, 160
handicapped people, 132
health, 10
heart failure, 78
height, 117, 118

helium, 89
hemangioma, viii, 36
hematomas, 47
hematuria, 45
hemiparesis, 43
hemoptysis, 41
hemorrhage, xiii, 8, 44, 50, 51, 153, 155, 160
hepatitis, 46
hepatocytes, 82
hepatoma, 73, 82, 102
herpes, xiii, 7, 36, 37, 39, 45, 46, 60, 110, 154, 155, 156, 157, 159, 163, 164
herpes simplex, 110
herpes virus, xiii, 7, 36, 37, 39, 46, 154, 155, 156, 157, 159, 163, 164
herpes zoster, 45, 60
heterosexuals, 155
histidine, 77, 128
histological examination, 14
histology, 31, 32, 87
history, 54, 155, 163
HIV, viii, xiii, xiv, 7, 35, 37, 38, 39, 41, 42, 44, 45, 46, 48, 51, 54, 56, 57, 58, 59, 60, 154, 155, 157, 158, 159, 160, 164
HIV test, 48
HIV/AIDS, 155, 164
HIV-1, 48
homelessness, 47
homocysteine, 83
homosexuals, 155
host, ix, 63, 64, 104
human, x, 7, 34, 36, 39, 46, 56, 58, 59, 66, 81, 83, 84, 93, 94, 98, 102, 103, 105, 107, 108, 109, 110, 120, 121, 122, 125, 126, 127, 128, 132, 136, 154, 156, 157
human body, 46, 127
human immunodeficiency virus, 56, 59, 154
hyaline, 3, 50, 51
hydrogels, x, 86, 96, 97, 98, 102, 110
hydrogen, 128
hyoid, 90, 101
hyperbilirubinemia, 78
hypernephroma, 47
hypothesis, 94, 128

hypothyroidism, 45
hypoxia, 94, 104, 127
hypoxia-inducible factor, 104

I

iatrogenic, 6, 36, 37, 44, 56
idiopathic, 36, 154
IFN, 111, 114, 119
IFNβ, 113
IFN-β, 111
IFN-β, 114
IFN-β, 119
ILAR, 122
ileum, xiv, 154, 156, 158
illumination, 125, 126, 127, 129, 136
image, 31, 32, 41, 135
image analysis, 31, 32
images, xiii, 41, 115, 118, 154
immersion, 126
immune response, 110, 111, 119
immune system, 37, 46
immunity, xi, 108
immunodeficiency, vii, 2, 48, 61, 155
immunogenicity, 111, 119
immunohistochemistry, 57
immunomodulatory, 56
immunoreactivity, 10
immunostimulatory, xi, 108, 119
immunosuppression, 40, 56, 103, 119, 155
immunosuppressive drugs, 30
immunosuppressive therapies, 7
immunotherapy, 55, 111, 114, 119
implants, viii, 2, 6
improvements, 46
in vitro, v, x, 79, 80, 85, 86, 90, 92, 93, 95, 96, 97, 102, 103, 105, 106, 111, 121, 125, 126, 127
in vivo, ix, 64, 79, 92, 93, 94, 95, 97, 101, 103, 105, 121, 122, 125, 126, 127, 137
indolent, 38, 46
induction, 111
infancy, 3
infarction, 8

infection, viii, xiii, xiv, 35, 37, 39, 44, 46, 47, 54, 56, 58, 60, 119, 154, 155, 157, 158, 159, 160, 162, 164
inflammation, 104
inflammatory cells, 50
infliximab, 56
informed consent, 112, 156
inguinal, 39
inhibition, 65, 66, 68, 71, 73, 74, 76, 78, 83, 84, 106, 110, 128, 136
inhibitor, 66, 74, 76, 77, 78, 103
injections, 110, 113, 115, 118, 119
injuries, 49, 52
injury, viii, 36, 73, 82
inoculation, 69
institutions, 28
insulin, 103
integration, 104
integrin, 95, 98, 105
integrins, 105
interface, 104
interferon, xi, 55, 61, 108, 111, 120, 121, 122
intervention, 142
intestinal tract, xiv, 154
intestine, 40
intravenously, 132
ions, 89, 100, 128
Iowa, 103, 127
ipsilateral, 118
irradiation, 18, 29, 90, 125, 127
isolation, 42
Israel, 32, 38, 58
issues, 117, 143
Italy, 1, 38, 58, 123, 139

J

Japan, 63, 123, 153, 155
jejunum, 41, 163
joints, vii, xi, 1, 9, 17, 124
jumping, 124

K

Kaposi sarcoma, 7, 37, 40, 41, 42, 48, 51, 54, 55, 59, 60, 61, 62, 154, 164
Kenya, 39
keratinocyte, 78
kidney, 45, 60, 162
kill, 90
knees, 5

L

labeling, 136
laboratory tests, 14
lactate dehydrogenase, 136
lactic acid, 136
laminectomy, 146
laparotomy, 61
laryngoscopy, 44
larynx, 44, 142
latency, 52
laws and regulations, 112
lead, x, xiv, 8, 29, 86, 142, 143, 147, 154
leakage, 128
learning, ix, 36
leiomyoma, 4
lesions, viii, xiii, xiv, 2, 8, 10, 11, 12, 17, 21, 23, 24, 32, 36, 38, 39, 40, 41, 42, 43, 44, 45, 46, 47, 48, 49, 51, 55, 56, 98, 113, 141, 146, 147, 153, 154, 155, 156, 157, 158, 160, 161
leukemia, 18, 66, 67, 81, 83
lice, 47
life quality, x, 86, 88, 89
light, 11, 22, 90, 125, 126, 127, 128, 129, 136
light beam, 127
lipids, 119
lipoma, 3, 8, 11
liposomes, 112, 122
liver, ix, xiv, 10, 48, 63, 64, 67, 68, 70, 71, 76, 154, 159
localization, 16, 24, 27, 42, 126
locus, 18

low risk, xi, xii, 124, 125, 133
lumbar spine, 43
lumen, 42
luminescence, 127
lung metastases, 29, 110, 121
lymph node, viii, xiii, xiv, 10, 11, 13, 17, 25, 35, 37, 38, 39, 40, 41, 48, 49, 51, 54, 57, 109, 118, 120, 153, 154, 155, 159, 164
lymphadenopathy, 24, 42, 47
lymphangioma, 38
lymphatic system, 48
lymphedema, 41
lymphocytes, 50, 51
lymphoma, 6, 20, 22, 37, 39, 54
lysosome, 126, 128

M

macrophages, 50, 51, 134
magnetic resonance imaging, 17, 147
magnetic resonance scanning, 143
majority, 9, 18, 21, 22, 41, 155
malabsorption, 41
malaise, 23
malaria, 134
malignancy, viii, 5, 6, 13, 20, 26, 35, 40, 41, 49, 94, 155, 160, 163
malignant melanoma, 111, 136
malignant tumors, vii, 1, 11, 19, 23, 24
management, xiii, 14, 17, 21, 29, 32, 33, 87, 88, 90, 97, 99, 140, 147, 148, 149, 151
mandible, 44, 118
mapping, 49
Maryland, 60
mass, viii, 2, 9, 10, 12, 21, 23, 28, 43, 44, 45, 113, 115
mastoid, 143
materials, 96, 105, 124, 126
matrix, 8, 19, 24, 86, 87, 102, 105
maxilla, 44, 118
median, xi, xiv, 5, 6, 13, 37, 38, 42, 108, 110, 120, 154, 158, 160
medical, 57, 157
medication, 112

medicine, 12, 32, 76, 78, 97, 105
Mediterranean, 36, 37, 38, 154, 165
melanoma, xi, 12, 44, 108, 110, 111, 114, 119, 120, 121, 122, 136
membranes, 80, 134
meninges, 42, 143, 147
mental health, ix, 36
messenger RNA, 125
metabolism, 37, 65, 77, 92
metalloproteinase, 106
metastasis, ix, 7, 12, 13, 22, 24, 25, 26, 28, 29, 32, 56, 59, 63, 64, 68, 70, 71, 80, 87, 88, 94, 95, 104, 109, 111, 115, 117, 126, 145, 146
metastatic disease, viii, 2, 22, 25, 104, 109, 110, 116, 117, 141, 146, 147
meter, 126
mice, vii, ix, 63, 64, 66, 67, 68, 70, 73, 77, 79, 82, 93, 128, 132, 134, 137
microorganisms, 134
microscope, 12, 50, 125, 126, 129
microscopy, 136
Middle East, 38
mitochondria, 125
mitosis, 51, 52
model system, x, 107
models, x, 86, 90, 92, 93, 94, 95, 96, 97, 102, 110
modifications, 103
molecular biology, 141
molecular pathology, 101
molecules, 94, 96
momentum, 110
monoclonal antibody, 51, 62
montelukast, 56
Moon, 106, 150
morbidity, 15, 42, 56, 142, 143, 147
Morocco, 58
morphogenesis, 98
morphology, 37, 49
mortality, 6, 30, 42, 46, 54, 94
mortality rate, 6
mosaic, 134
Moses, 104
MRI, 11, 12, 14, 17, 24, 43, 45

MTS, 115
mucosa, viii, 36, 48, 156
mucous membranes, 40
multiple myeloma, 17
muscles, viii, xi, 35, 124, 126
musculoskeletal system, 44, 60
mutagen, 132
mutant, 73, 82
mutation, 18
mutilation, 145
myositis, 3

N

Na^+, 82
nasopharynx, 143
nausea, 41
necrosis, 8, 90
neon, 89
neoplasm, xii, 9, 62, 88, 94, 139
nerve, 3, 6, 23, 43, 78, 143
Netherlands, 104
neuroblastoma, 22, 24
neurotoxicity, 73
nevus, 48
Nigeria, 39
nitrogen, 124
nodes, 13, 38, 39, 145, 159
nodules, 24, 37, 38, 41, 42, 44, 47, 49, 50, 69, 103, 156
North America, 38
NSAIDs, 56
nuclei, 19, 22
nucleic acid, 110, 133
nucleolus, 125
nutrition, 92, 96

O

obstruction, viii, xiii, 21, 36, 41, 43, 45, 153, 155, 160
occult blood, xiii, 48, 154, 158, 159
old age, 21
operations, 141

opportunities, 109, 148
oral cavity, xiv, 40, 59, 154, 157, 159
orbit, 44, 150
organ, xiv, 40, 44, 45, 49, 57, 81, 119, 154, 155, 159
organelles, 125
organs, viii, xiv, 7, 35, 37, 40, 46, 48, 49, 57, 154, 159, 163
osmotic pressure, 78
ossification, 24
osteochondroma, 21
osteogenic sarcoma, xii, 140
osteoma, 20
osteotomy, 117
ovarian cancer, 97, 106
overproduction, 94
overweight, 118
oxygen, 92, 102, 128, 134

P

p53, 6, 12, 34
paclitaxel, 55
pain, viii, xi, 2, 19, 21, 23, 29, 41, 42, 43, 44, 45, 108, 109, 114, 115, 116, 117, 118, 158
palate, 40, 44, 54, 118
palliative, 15, 16, 29, 115, 118, 120, 142, 147
parasites, 125, 134
parathyroid, 106
parathyroid hormone, 106
parenchyma, 41
pathogenesis, 6, 7, 41, 155
pathogens, 46
pathologist, 12, 161
pathology, ix, 36, 59, 60, 164
pathways, 99
PCR, 73, 158, 159, 160
pelvis, 5, 9, 21, 44, 86, 88
perforation, xiii, 153, 155, 160, 161
perfusion, 16, 33
periosteum, 19
peripheral blood, 164
peritoneum, 127

permeability, 66, 78
peroxide, 83
PET scan, 14
pH, 101, 125, 126, 128, 134, 135, 136
pharynx, 142
phenotypes, 94, 95, 103, 105
Philadelphia, 29
photolithography, 96
photons, 89, 100
photopolymerization, 105
physical activity, 133
physiology, 94, 105
pilot study, 98, 120, 121
plaque, 38, 49
plasma cells, 50
plasma membrane, 136
plasmid, 110, 112, 119
platform, 91, 93, 102, 106
platinum, 83
pleural effusion, 42
plexus, 43
PM, 143, 144, 150
pneumocystis pneumonia, 162
pneumonia, 42, 46
polydimethylsiloxane, 102
polymerization, 96
polypectomy, 61
pons, 42
positron, 11
positron emission tomography (PET), 11, 14, 25, 157
preservation, 133
primary tumor, xi, 13, 25, 40, 69, 108, 109, 151
private practice, 120
prognosis, viii, ix, 2, 8, 13, 21, 26, 29, 31, 32, 40, 57, 63, 64, 90, 125, 146, 147
proliferation, 37, 51, 91, 104, 106, 157
promoter, 111
prostate cancer, 102
protection, 83
protein family, 84
proteins, 32, 96
proton pump inhibitors, 136
protons, 89, 100, 128

pumps, 66
purpura, 47
pyogenic, 44, 47

Q

quality of life, xi, 14, 64, 108, 111, 113, 116, 118, 120, 124, 132

R

race, 18
radiation, vii, viii, xi, 1, 2, 6, 8, 9, 14, 15, 16, 18, 22, 27, 28, 29, 33, 34, 45, 55, 87, 89, 100, 105, 108, 109, 120, 122, 127, 135, 136, 143, 150
radiation therapy, vii, xi, 1, 15, 18, 22, 27, 28, 29, 33, 34, 55, 100, 108, 109, 122, 150
radio, 89, 97, 127, 135
radiography, viii, 2, 17, 19, 22, 24, 115, 116, 117
radioresistance, 97
radiotherapy, x, xii, xiii, 6, 13, 15, 16, 17, 21, 28, 29, 33, 86, 88, 89, 100, 140, 141, 142, 143, 144, 145, 146, 147
radius, 44, 116, 118
reactions, 64, 65, 66, 76
receptors, 73, 91
reciprocal translocation, 8
recommendations, iv, 17
reconstruction, xi, 27, 33, 88, 124
recovery, 46, 78, 115, 124
rectum, xiv, 30, 154, 156, 158
recurrence, x, xi, xii, 11, 12, 14, 15, 16, 17, 22, 25, 27, 28, 86, 87, 88, 99, 108, 111, 117, 118, 119, 120, 124, 125, 129, 131, 133
red blood cells, 50
regression, 55, 56, 115
rehabilitation, 15
rejection, 111
relapses, 146
remission, xi, 108, 113, 116, 120, 151

remodelling, 103
reproductive age, 28
researchers, 89
resection, xi, xii, xiii, 14, 27, 29, 33, 88, 89, 99, 117, 124, 132, 135, 140, 141, 142, 143, 145, 146
residual disease, 111, 142
residuals, 141
resistance, ix, x, 63, 64, 66, 74, 75, 84, 86, 95, 97, 104, 111, 136
resolution, 11, 101, 115, 126, 147
response, 11, 16, 25, 26, 28, 37, 55, 62, 92, 97, 98, 104, 105, 110, 113, 115, 118, 134, 144, 163
restoration, 115, 118
retardation, 134
reticulum, ix, 63, 64, 80, 81, 125
retinoblastoma, 18
ribonucleic acid, 133, 134
ribosomal RNA, 125
risk, xii, 6, 8, 14, 15, 16, 18, 27, 28, 34, 47, 54, 109, 124, 132, 143, 160, 164
risk factors, 18
risks, x, xiii, 15, 86, 88, 140
RNAs, 106, 125, 128
roots, 23
routes, 157
rural areas, 38
Rwanda, 163

S

sacrum, 31
safety, xi, 76, 108, 111, 114, 120
saliva, 155
salivary glands, viii, 35, 45
sampling error, 141
scapula, 98
scar tissue, 6
sclerosis, 24
seafood, 77
secrete, 110
secretion, xi, 44, 108, 111, 125, 127
seed, 94
semen, 155

sensitivity, ix, 12, 36, 63, 64, 67, 74, 76, 83, 92
sequencing, 28
serum, 23, 34, 119
sex, xiv, 37, 154, 155, 158, 159, 160
sexual behavior, 158
sexual contact, 155
shape, 24
shortness of breath, 41
showing, 115
side effects, 15, 119
sigmoid colon, 156
signaling pathway, 91, 101
signalling, 104
signs, ix, 7, 36, 39, 42, 57, 115, 117
silver, 47
simulation, 128
sinuses, 143, 149, 150, 151
siRNA, 106
skeletal muscle, 7, 44, 77
skeleton, 17, 44
skin, vii, viii, xiii, xiv, 1, 4, 22, 23, 27, 35, 36, 37, 38, 39, 40, 41, 42, 45, 47, 48, 49, 50, 54, 55, 56, 125, 153, 154, 155, 157, 159, 161, 162, 164
smooth muscle cells, 7
sodium, 83
soft tissue sarcomas, vii, xii, 1, 30, 31, 32, 33, 140, 149, 150
soft tissue tumors, 3, 7, 13, 126
solid tumors, 101
solution, 96, 126, 129, 132
South Africa, 37
South America, 38
species, 109, 110
spinal cord, 43, 44
spindle, 3, 4, 8, 9, 19, 26, 50, 51, 52, 156
spine, 22, 43, 88, 89, 100
stabilization, 113
state, x, 86, 101, 110, 148
sterile, 111
sternum, 44
stimulus, 111
stomach, xiv, 41, 154, 156, 158, 161, 163
stress, 78, 128

stridor, 42, 43
stroma, 9, 19, 50, 96, 104
stromal cells, 9
structure, 22, 56, 74, 78, 82, 92
subacute, 11
subcutaneous injection, 112
subcutaneous tissue, 38, 45, 50, 60, 93
submucosa, 157
substrate, 74, 78, 82
suicide, vii, xi, 108, 110, 111, 114, 115, 117, 118, 119, 120, 121
Sun, 104
suppression, 66, 69, 74, 80, 91
surgical intervention, xi, 12, 108
surgical removal, xi, 29, 87, 108, 118, 120
surgical resection, xiii, 16, 28, 29, 88, 109, 140, 142, 143, 144, 146, 151
surveillance, 30
survival, xi, xii, xiii, 12, 13, 15, 22, 26, 27, 28, 29, 39, 42, 55, 56, 87, 89, 90, 99, 105, 106, 108, 109, 111, 119, 120, 121, 122, 131, 140, 143, 144, 146, 147, 164
survival rate, xi, 22, 26, 42, 87, 89, 90, 108, 109, 120, 122, 131, 146
survivors, 16, 29, 132
susceptibility, vii, 1, 73, 82
swelling, viii, 2, 19, 21, 23, 45, 115, 116, 118, 128
symptoms, vii, viii, ix, xiii, xiv, 2, 7, 17, 23, 36, 48, 49, 54, 57, 89, 117, 154, 158, 159, 160, 161
syndrome, 6, 18, 46, 47, 48, 56, 60, 61, 62
synovitis, 23
synthesis, 74, 76, 83

T

target, 90, 91, 103
technical assistance, 120
techniques, viii, xiii, 2, 25, 27, 140, 141, 147
telangiectasia, 48
telencephalon, 73
tendon sheath, 3
tendons, 9, 124
testing, 48
TGF, 104
therapeutic interventions, 101
therapeutic targets, 90, 97, 101, 105
therapy, vii, viii, x, xi, xii, 2, 9, 14, 15, 16, 21, 22, 23, 27, 28, 31, 32, 33, 37, 40, 46, 55, 56, 59, 61, 62, 64, 67, 80, 89, 90, 91, 93, 100, 101, 102, 108, 110, 111, 119, 121, 124, 127, 133, 135, 140, 143, 148, 149, 150, 155, 160
third dimension, 102
thoracotomy, 29, 146
thorax, 42
thrombocytopenia, 61
thrush, 54
thymoma, 4
thyroid gland, 45
tibia, 19, 24, 44, 94
tissue, vii, viii, x, xi, xii, xiii, 1, 2, 4, 7, 9, 10, 12, 14, 15, 19, 21, 22, 24, 25, 27, 29, 30, 31, 32, 33, 34, 45, 47, 50, 52, 73, 86, 88, 89, 93, 94, 95, 96, 97, 98, 99, 105, 106, 108, 118, 126, 127, 130, 131, 135, 137, 139, 141, 142, 143, 154
tissue perfusion, 95
tourniquet, 16
toxicity, 15, 74, 76, 119, 132, 142
trachea, 42
traits, 105
transcription, 6, 32
transduction, 122
transfer RNA, 125, 134
transformation, 6
translocation, 9, 22, 26
transmission, 73
transplant, 36, 37, 40, 44, 45, 49, 155, 162
transplant recipients, 37, 162
transplantation, 7, 28, 33, 40, 60, 93, 94
transport, 65, 67, 71, 72, 73, 74, 75, 76, 78, 80, 81, 82, 84, 91
transport processes, 65
trauma, 38, 45
traumatic events, viii, 2
treatment methods, 91
trial, xi, 100, 108, 111, 112, 120, 135

Index

trisomy, 10
tuberculosis, 46
tumor cells, 8, 14, 22, 66, 69, 71, 73, 74, 76, 77, 78, 79, 93, 94, 104, 110
tumor growth, 68, 94, 111, 127
tumor metastasis, 70
tumor necrosis factor, 16
tumor progression, 103
tumorigenesis, 94
tumors, x, 2, 5, 6, 7, 8, 9, 10, 11, 13, 16, 17, 18, 19, 21, 22, 24, 25, 26, 27, 30, 31, 34, 38, 39, 41, 51, 52, 62, 66, 69, 71, 79, 87, 98, 99, 104, 105, 107, 110, 114, 119, 121, 125, 131, 134, 135, 136, 149, 151
tumour growth, 105
tumours, xii, xiii, 32, 98, 99, 101, 102, 104, 139, 140, 143, 144, 145, 147, 148
Tyrosine, 103

U

UK, 33
ulcer, 156
ulna, 44, 116
ultrasound, 25, 32, 58, 60
United States (USA), vii, 1, 5, 17, 58, 82, 85, 97, 112, 127, 132, 136, 164
ureter, 60
urinalysis, 115, 116
urinary retention, 45
uterus, 7, 30

V

vaccine, 111, 113, 115, 118, 119, 120, 121
valine, 77
variables, 26, 34, 39
variations, 96
vascular endothelial growth factor (VEGF), 41
vascularization, 11, 94
VEGF expression, 104
vehicles, 110
vein, 21
vertebrae, 43, 44
vessels, xi, 7, 51, 56, 69, 124, 164
viral gene, 121
viral infection, vii, 2, 6
viscera, 22, 47, 49, 54
visualization, 11, 129
vomiting, 41

W

Washington, 98
weight loss, 54
Western blot, 73
wheezing, 42
World Health Organization (WHO), 1, 3, 7, 19, 20, 94, 99, 132
wound infection, 121

9/13

3 4351 00030406 0

MILLVILLE PUBLIC LIBRARY
210 BUCK ST.
MILLVILLE, NJ 08332

07/18/2013